People... not Patients

People... not Patients

A Source Book for Living with Inflammatory Bowel Disease

Edited by: **Penny Steiner, M.P.H.**
Director, Research and Education
National Foundation for Ileitis & Colitis

Peter A. Banks, M.D.
Chief, Division of Gastroenterology
St. Elizabeth's Hospital, Boston

Daniel H. Present, M.D.
Associate Clinical Professor of Gastroenterology
Mt. Sinai Medical Center, New York

Graphics: Chase/Temkin & Associates
Printing: S & R Litho, Inc.
Index: June G. Rosenberg
Typesetting: JCH Graphics, Ltd.

The National Foundation for
Ileitis & Colitis

National Headquarters: 444 Park Avenue South, New York, N.Y. 10016 Tel: (212) 685-3440

Library of Congress Catalog Card Number 85–62308

First Printing, October 1985

ISBN 0–9615495–0–5

Contributors

Harvey Arbesman, M.D.
State University of New York
Buffalo, New York

Peter A. Banks, M.D.
St. Elizabeth's Hospital
Boston, Massachusetts

L. Kay Bartholomew, M.P.H.
Texas Children's Hospital
Houston, Texas

Joel J. Bauer, M.D.
Mount Sinai Medical Center
New York, New York

Marjorie Beck, R.N.
Abington Memorial Hospital
Abington, Pennsylvania

Philip S. Bentlif, M.D.
Kelsey-Seybold Clinic
Houston, Texas

Donald P. Binder
United Ostomy Association
Los Angeles, California

Debra C. Broadwell, R.N., E.T., Ph.D.
Emory University
Atlanta, Georgia

Danita Czyzewski, Ph.D.
Texas Children's Hospital
Houston, Texas

Frances J. Dory
New York City Self-Help Clearinghouse
Brooklyn, New York

George D. Ferry, M.D.
Texas Children's Hospital
Houston, Texas

Henry D. Janowitz, M.D.
Mount Sinai Medical Center
New York, New York

Marvin Kaplan, M.D.
Lenox Hill Hospital
New York, New York

Leonard A. Katz, M.D.
State University of New York
Buffalo, New York

Barbara S. Kirschner, M.D.
University of Chicago
Chicago, Illinois

Marvin Lieberman, Ph.D.
New York Academy of Medicine
New York, New York

Michigan Chapter
National Foundation for Ileitis and Colitis
Detroit, Michigan

Michael L. Miller, C.L.U.
New York, New York

Lee Anne Moses, R.N., B.S.N.
Texas Children's Hospital
Houston, Texas

Daniel H. Present, M.D.
Mount Sinai Hospital
New York, New York

Jane W. Present, M.A.
New York, New York

Arvey I. Rogers, M.D.
Veterans Administration Medical Center
Miami, Florida

David Roseman, M.D.
Scripps Memorial Hospital
La Jolla, California

Milton Singer, M.D.
St. Barnabas Medical Center
Livingston, New Jersey

Howard M. Spiro, M.D.
Yale-New Haven Medical Center
New Haven, Connecticut

Penny Steiner, M.P.H.
National Foundation for Ileitis and Colitis
New York, New York

Stephen P. Stowe, M.D.
Genesee Hospital
Rochester, New York

Marjorie M. Sutton, M.S., R.D.
University of Chicago
Chicago, Illinois

Maurice J. Zimmerman, M.D.
Mount Sinai Medical Center
New York, New York

Contents

Preface

People with inflammatory bowel disease are patients only *some* of the time. The rest of the time they have jobs to do, hobbies to pursue, people to love and care for, families to raise.

As recently as 10 or 20 years ago, it was not unusual for people with Crohn's disease or ulcerative colitis to blame themselves for having diseases they barely understood. All this has changed. Today, these same people are gathering strength from each other, becoming knowledgeable about the medical and surgical treatment of IBD, starting support and hospital visitation groups, and learning about their rights within the health care system.

People with inflammatory bowel disease are patients only some of the time.

In planning the content of this book, we decided that we wanted to give people with IBD the tools to become advocates in their own behalf. To do that they would need a source book with sufficient information to help them understand the diseases, learn about their legal rights, and begin to fight back. We sought the help of many individuals who share this philosophy and purpose. There were physicians, nurse specialists, enterostomal therapists, people with the diseases, people with ostomies, family members and friends.

We wish to thank the many people who have contributed material for this book, and those special people with IBD who let us tell their stories so that others could find inspiration. In addition, we want to thank Andrea Haber, Terry Jennings, and Sharon Walsh who helped provide some of the material in Chapter 6; Marla Singer Gellerman who helped type and proofread the manuscript; June Rosenberg who prepared the index; Roy Temkin of Chase/Temkin & Associates, and everyone at S&R Litho, Inc. for producing the book. Special thanks must go to Marjorie Merrick who assisted in every phase of the project and provided us with her unique blend of humor and common sense along the way.

In addition, we want to thank Sandoz, Inc. for making it possible for us to print this book. Through their generosity, we will be able to reach many thousands of people with IBD who need the information contained in these pages. Lastly, we wish to thank our readers, the people with IBD, their families and friends. We hope you will learn as much from this book as we have learned from you.

Penny Steiner
Peter A. Banks
Daniel H. Present

Foreword

Howard M. Spiro, M.D.

Until the long-sought cure is found, inflammatory bowel disease remains a life-long, *transfiguring* disease of uncertain cause with inescapable and humiliating symptoms whose therapy has not changed very much in thirty years. To be sure, each year new triumphs in the understanding of IBD are reported, but on the whole, what we know of IBD does not seem so very much different from that of my medical youth. Then we learned that "Bargen's bacillus" was the cause of some cases of inflammatory bowel disease, that allergy to an agent probably determined the response and that a vaccine might be helpful. The current immunological paradigm of T cells and B cells, suppressor and killer cells complicates the suggestion that some infectious agent gains entrance to the gastrointestinal tract and there, depending upon immunological responses, causes Crohn's disease or maybe even ulcerative colitis. This is not so very different from the 1940 model.

From the patient's standpoint, advances in therapy make for little optimism. Physicians use approximately the same drugs in the management of IBD today as we did in the late 1940's. Sulfasalazine was first used about 1942 and it was in 1948-49 that we began to use steroids. There have been some steps forward since then: metronidazole, immunosuppressive therapy, intravenous hyperalimentation, and the like, but the major standard therapies were in use more than a quarter of a century ago. In how many fields must such a confession still be made?

The symptoms of IBD have little redeeming value. Physicians, theologians and philosophers have written a great deal about pain, about putting up with it, about finding lessons in it, but who has written of the affirmative qualities of diarrhea? So far as I know, no philosopher has found lessons for life in having to rush off to the toilet, though many have talked of the lessons of pain. For our patients, the symptoms of IBD are inescapable and humiliating. Pain can be ignored, borne, or put off in a way that diarrhea makes quite inescapable. Physicians should ask their patients what inflammatory bowel disease has done to them and how it has affected their daily lives. They might be surprised at the answers.

If the cure for IBD has eluded us for so long, gastroenterologists should pay at least as much attention to care as they do to the diagnostic apparatus. In that regard, it is important to keep in mind the distinctions between *disease* and *illness*. Disease is biomedically detectable, quantifiable, physical and structural. It is what the doctor sees, what the image depicts, on ultrasonography, barium enema, or endoscopy. Illness is the subjective component, the response to the disease.

It is the feeling that goes along with a disease, it is the patient's voice. Too often the meanings of disease and illness are mixed and the terms are used as synonyms. Not too long ago, gastroenterologists had so little they could do *to* their patients that they used to spend time *with* them. To look at IBD from the patient's standpoint is to look at 1) disability ("Where's the toilet? Can I go to work? Play tennis?"); 2) anxiety ("Why another sigmoidoscopy? What is eating at me?"); 3) foreboding ("Do I have cancer? Do I need an ileostomy?"); 4) suffering ("I am so sick of the doctors.") I simply want to emphasize how different are disease and illness and that gastroenterologists spend too much time on the objective findings and not enough time with the patient and his/her concerns.

Inflammatory bowel disease is much like cancer: it transforms life. Once you have cancer, you are never the same person again, and are never free from fear of recurrence. In a real sense, you are transfigured, you become a "cancer patient" not just Mr. X or Mrs. Y or Miss Z. The person who gets inflammatory bowel disease, too, is transfigured and from then on must devote a considerable amount of energy to dealing with the disease. A testimony to the weight of that disease is the very success of such a foundation as the National Foundation for Ileitis and Colitis. There were no groups of "concerned ulcer patients" because even before current therapy, having an ulcer did not really change your life. For the person with IBD, diarrhea is an ever-present threat, cancer is a long-term concern, and loneliness, anxiety, dependency, depression and guilt are a challenge and often a daily frustration.

These are matters we should talk about more. When they could cure few diseases, physicians were healers of illness. Today, physicians order x-rays and other tests, insert scopes, and give pills, but healing comes from technical skills and they would be embarrassed to think that their words had power. Yes, we must do tests, but we should also take time to listen. Sometimes we may find that the healing power of listening and talking proves almost as great as that which comes from steroids and sulfasalazine. Our patients want to be independent and we should emphasize self-management. But, just as important, we should use words as well as drugs.

Understanding Your Illness

1 About Inflammatory Bowel Disease

The diseases we call Crohn's disease and ulcerative colitis have been given the convenient label "inflammatory bowel disease" (IBD) as if to emphasize their similiarities and minimize their differences. True, there are differences: Crohn's disease may affect any part of the bowel from mouth to anus while ulcerative colitis attacks only the colon; Crohn's disease involves the full thickness of bowel wall while ulcerative colitis inflames only the inner surface lining; ulcerative colitis is permanently cured by surgery while Crohn's disease is not. Crohn's disease has increased dramatically in incidence over the past few decades while ulcerative colitis has remained stable. These are important differences, but at the present time, the similarities between the two diseases appear to overshadow the differences.

At the present time, the similarities between the two forms of IBD appear to overshadow the differences.

Both types of IBD occur predominantly in Western or developed countries of the world, especially Scandinavia, England, Western Europe, Israel and the United States. Conversely, IBD is rarely detected in peoples of Africa, Asia and parts of South America, areas of poor sanitation and lower nutritional standards. Jews in particular have an unusually high incidence of both diseases (four to five times normal), while blacks and orientals have a relatively low incidence. Although all ages are at risk for IBD, the high risk age group for both diseases is ages 12 to 40, with equal division among sexes. A full 10 percent are young people under the age of 18. Crohn's disease and ulcerative colitis tend to cluster in some families, although a specific genetic pattern has not been identified. About 20-25 percent of people with IBD have one or more relatives with either disease.

The purpose of this introductory chapter is to summarize current knowledge about both forms of IBD, with special emphasis on the nature of the inflammatory process they have in common, and on the search for an immune or infectious etiology.

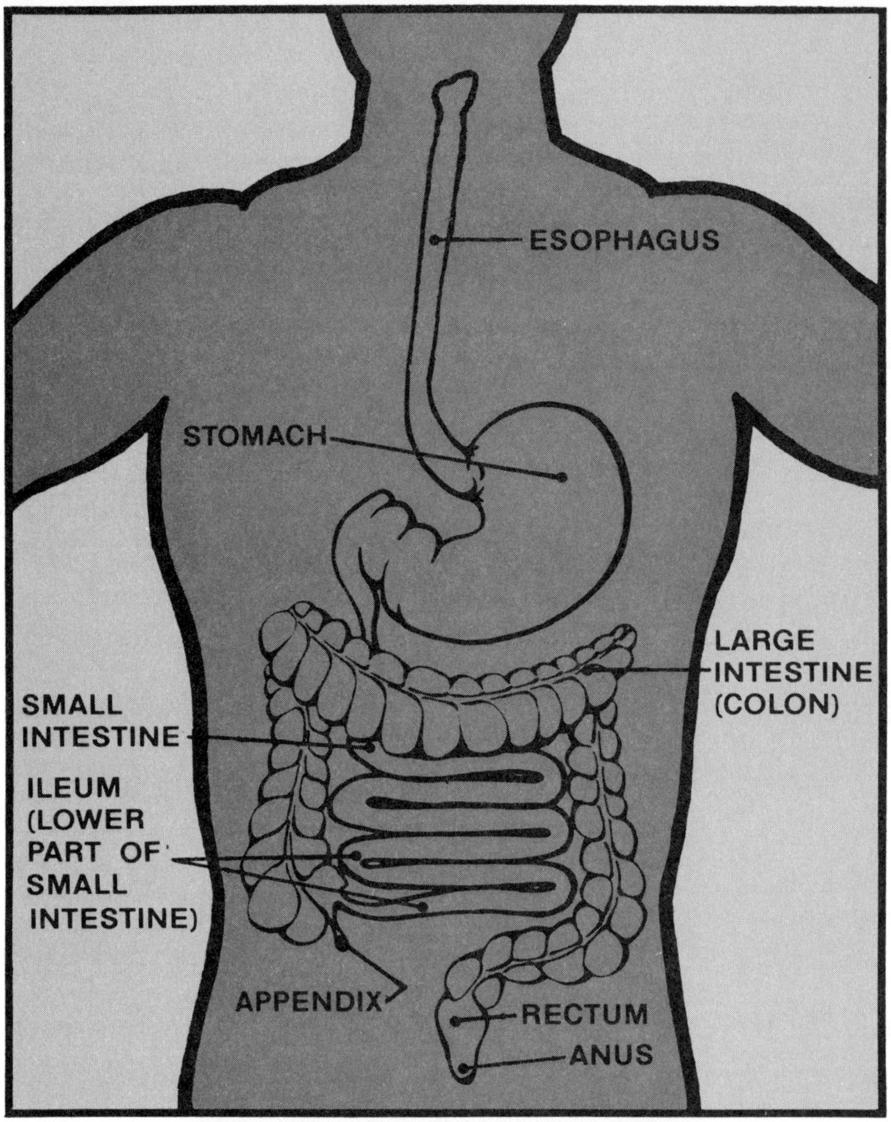

Diagram of the gastrointestinal tract

About Ulcerative Colitis

Although they are "first cousins," there are important differences between ulcerative colitis and Crohn's disease. Ulcerative colitis attacks the large bowel (colon) exclusively and only the inner lining membranes (mucosa and submucosa). The inflammation almost always involves the rectum and extends backward through the colon, but never extends beyond the junction of the large and small bowel, an anatomic landmark called the ileocecal valve. Involvement of the colon is continuous, never patchy. Superficial ulcers occur and the bowel lining becomes congested and friable, bleeding easily on slight contact.

People with ulcerative colitis feel a frequent need to defecate since the inflamed rectum is repeatedly distended with liquid stool. Characteristically, the bowel movements are frequent but small in volume and crampy abdominal pain with defecation urgency is common. Since the inner lining is ulcerated and friable, rectal bleeding is very common. The need to have frequent bowel movements may interfere with sleep and interrupt meals, work, school, athletics, and the enjoyment of life. In severe cases where the entire colon is involved, systemic symptoms such as fever, muscle aching, sweats, and impaired appetite may occur. Blood loss may lead to anemia. The course of ulcerative colitis is usually chronic with periods of spontaneous healing (remission) and exacerbation (flare-ups). With medication and appropriate management, complete healing of ulcerations often occurs and the lining of the colon may appear entirely normal again. Relapses can occur quickly or take many years.

Twenty-five percent of cases of ulcerative colitis involve only the rectum and left colon (distal colitis) and symptoms are therefore less severe. When inflammation is confined to the rectum, it is called ulcerative proctitis.

In ulcerative proctitis, the symptoms are usually mild and well-tolerated. The disease usually remains localized in the rectum for years, and only occasionally progresses upward to other parts of the colon.

When medical treatment fails to control the symptoms of ulcerative colitis, surgical removal of the colon may be necessary. The conventional surgical approach for many years has been total proctocolectomy (removal of the entire colon and the rectum) and creation of an ileostomy. However, in some medical centers newer surgical procedures (continent ileostomy, ileoanal anastomosis) are available which preserve continence and make the wearing of an external appliance unnecessary. Removal of colon and rectum is a permanent cure for ulcerative colitis.

About Crohn's Disease

Crohn's disease (also known as regional enteritis) was confused with intestinal tuberculosis for many years until Crohn, Ginzburg and Oppenheimer described its characteristic features in a classic paper in 1932. It is now recognized as a major intestinal illness in the western world and its incidence seems to be steadily increasing.

The inflammation of Crohn's disease, in contrast to ulcerative colitis, involves the full thickness of the bowel wall rather than just the inner surface. It was originally thought that Crohn's disease involved only the lower small bowel or ileum. Later, it became evident that all parts of the digestive tract, including the esophagus, stomach, duodenum, and colon, as well as the small bowel, could be involved. On a microscopic level, certain blood cells aggregate together to form a characteristic cell cluster called a granuloma. Granulomas are fairly specific for Crohn's disease and facilitate its identification.

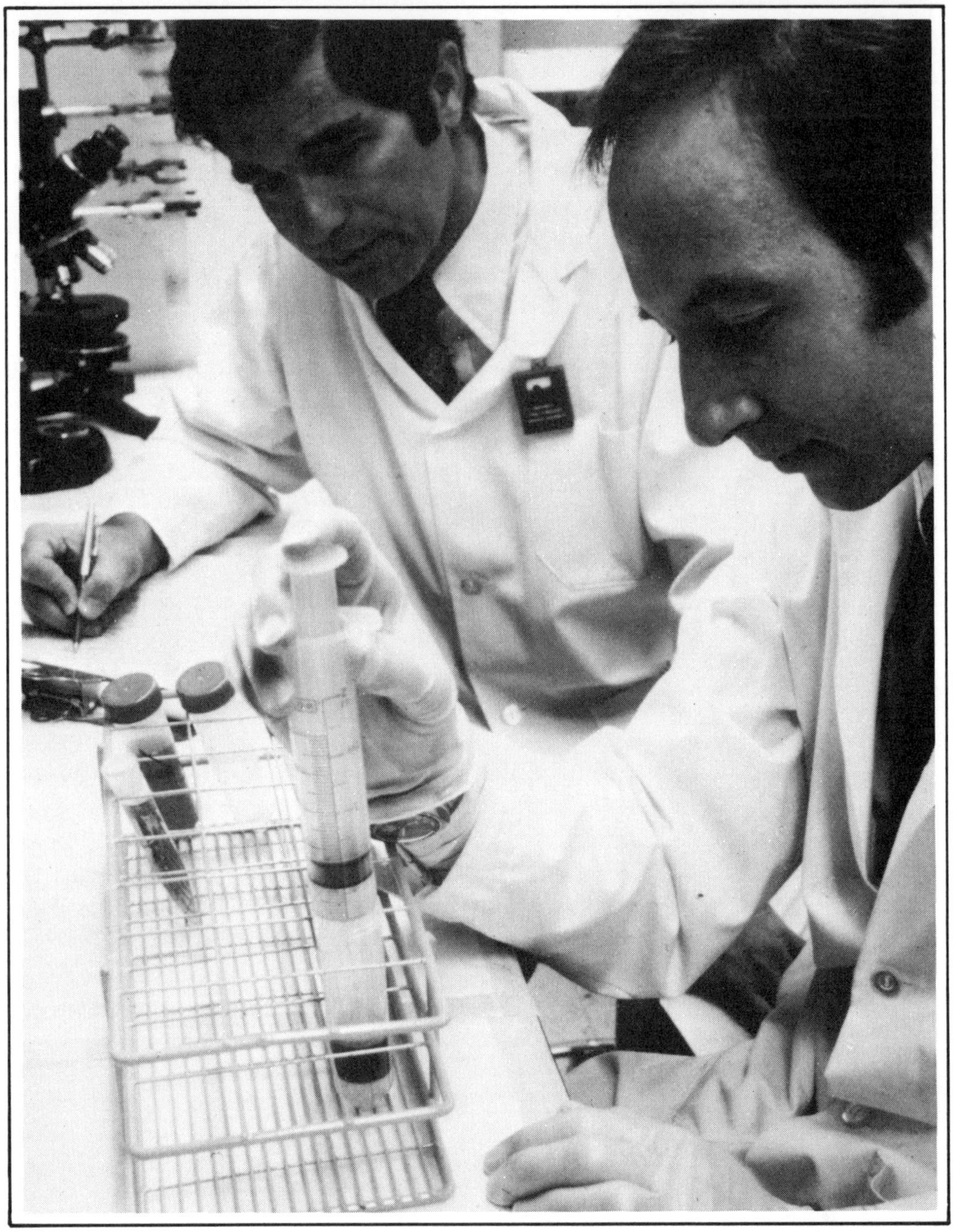

Perianal complications are very common in Crohn's disease and may be the first symptom, often appearing years before any intestinal problems. These include non-healing fissures, fistulas (abnormal channels around the anus), localized abscesses, and hemorrhoids.

People with Crohn's disease usually experience recurrent abdominal pain, and may have persistent non-bloody diarrhea (although stools can be normal). Fever, weakness and weight loss eventually occur. Because of the gradual onset of these symptoms, the disease is often overlooked or misdiagnosed, especially in children and adolescents. When recurrent pain is in the right lower portion of the abdomen, appendicitis may be suspected. Sometimes, extraintestinal manifestations such as skin eruptions and joint pains dominate the clinical picture and delay the diagnosis. The symptoms of Crohn's disease are so varied that each person can appear with different manifestations.

The course of Crohn's disease is characterized by periods of remission and exacerbation. Some people may have no symptoms for years, while others have chronic problems. However, even after successful medical and surgical therapy, the relapse rate is high, probably at least 75-80 percent. As a result, surgery is not considered a cure for Crohn's disease and is delayed until medical treatment has failed or complications occur.

The Inflammatory Response in IBD

Crohn's disease and ulcerative colitis have one very important feature in common—inflammation of the bowel wall. This inflammation follows the basic pattern of all types of inflammation in the body, but has some unique features.

The inflammatory response is the special way in which the body's immune system rallies to attack infecting or damaging agents. The affected area becomes warm, reddened, painful and swollen, and surrounding blood vessels become congested. "Inflammatory cells"—lymphocytes, leukocytes, mast cells and macrophages—migrate to the inflamed area. While attacking the invaders, these cells release powerful chemicals which also act as chemical "messengers" circulating in the blood to attract more inflammatory cells to the site.

Inflammation in the intestine has several hallmarks. In addition to the swelling, redness and pain, there is damage to the inner lining (mucosa), creating a break in the protective mucosal barrier. Ulcerations form, and normal cells and tissues may be exposed to intestinal bacteria and their harmful products as well as to enzymes released by the inflammatory cells. Blood and tissue fluid may leak from the intestinal wall, showing up as diarrhea or blood in the stool. The response by the body's inflammatory cells may cause even more damage than would have been caused by the original antigens (foreign substances such as bacteria, viruses, or chemicals). In this case the immune response is "out of control" or self-perpetuating.

The inflammatory response is also blamed for the so-called "systemic" manifestations of both types of IBD. These include joint pains, inflammation of the skin and eyes, and rare complications involving the liver and bile ducts.

A Possible Immune Cause

Some scientists feel that the immune response observed in IBD is a chronic state of inflammation, initiated by an unknown antigen and perpetuated by constant leakage of bacterial products through the wounded bowel wall. Others suggest that the inflammatory cells are reacting to the IBD patient's own tissues as if they were foreign, a process we know as autoimmunity. At the very least, we do know that certain specific disturbances have been found in persons with IBD. These findings do not prove an immune origin for IBD, but they do raise important questions which need to be answered. Are the immune disturbances seen in IBD patients the cause of the ailment, or are they an exaggerated response to an offending agent we have not yet located? If IBD is found to be caused by an infectious agent, isn't there still a disturbance in the immune response that prevents some people from overcoming the infection and subjects them to a chronic disease that lasts a lifetime?

The Search for an Infectious Agent

The search for an infectious agent in Crohn's disease and ulcerative colitis is complicated by the presence of a vast number and variety of microorganisms in normal human intestine. In the colon, for example, for every gram of stool there are an estimated one billion bacteria! Most of these bacteria carry out essential functions such as the breakdown of food and the production of certain essential vitamins. Finding a pathogenic or disease-causing organism—either a virus or bacterium—among such a crowded field has proved a formidable task for microbiologists and virologists over the past few decades.

Most recently, interest centers around a previously unrecognized species of mycobacterium which has been isolated from the intestines of several patients with Crohn's disease. This organism appears to cause a Crohn's-like illness in goats, but it will be some time before we know its role, if any, in IBD in humans.

Much has been learned about the patterns of inflammatory bowel disease in the past 50 years, not all of which could be contained within this chapter. Even though the causal agents have not yet been identified, people with IBD are capable of leading long, useful and often comfortable lives with careful medical and surgical management. Hopefully, expanding research programs, such as those sponsored by the National Foundation for Ileitis and Colitis, will lead to the identification of the offending agents and to the eventual eradication of this group of diseases. In the meantime, it is necessary to learn as much as possible about IBD, the demands it makes on our living patterns, and the ways we can learn to cope with those demands. This is the reason for this book.

For Further Information...

***The Crohn's Disease and Ulcerative Colitis Fact Book*, edited by Peter A. Banks, M.D., Daniel H. Present, M.D., and Penny Steiner, M.P.H. New York: Charles Scribner's Sons, 1983. (When purchased through the National Foundation for Ileitis and Colitis, all proceeds from the sale of this book are used to fund research and education programs of NFIC.)**

2

A Primer Of Diagnostic Procedures And Laboratory Tests In IBD

The physician relies on a variety of diagnostic procedures and laboratory tests in order to confirm a suspected diagnosis of inflammatory bowel disease. These tests can be categorized as follows: (1) blood and urine tests; (2) stool examinations; (3) radiologic procedures; and (4) endoscopic procedures. The physician is likely to use many of these same tests and procedures to assess the progress of the patient with IBD.

The purpose of this chapter is to tell you more about these particular procedures and tests as they relate to the diagnosis and management of IBD. When you finish reading the chapter, you should have a better understanding of:

- why a particular test has been selected;
- what the test results can and cannot tell about diagnosis and/or response to therapy;
- what you might expect in preparing for diagnostic procedures;
- how you might feel during the performance of radiologic and endoscopic examinations.

Blood and Urine Tests

For the most part, there is no preparation for these tests other than fasting for such tests as blood sugar or triglyceride (blood fat) determinations. A urine sample collected for purposes of culturing should be done under aseptic (clean) circumstances. The physician or nurse will instruct you on the proper method.

The **complete blood count** includes the hemoglobin, hematocrit, white blood cell count and a determination of the types of white blood cells making up the total count (the differential). The hemoglobin and hematocrit determine if anemia is present. There are techniques available which help to determine the cause of anemia, i.e. loss of blood, vitamin deficiency, or destruction of red blood cells (RBC's). The white blood cell (WBC) count and differential provide information about the degree of activity of an inflammatory reaction and whether or not infection is present. The WBC count is usually increased when active inflammation and/or infection are present. Corticosteroids also increase the white blood cell count. When significant inflammation and/or infection are present, younger white blood cells called "stab" or juvenile forms appear; this is reported usually as a "left shift." The **platelet count,** which measures cells involved in the clotting of blood, is usually raised above normal in the presence of active inflammation and/or infection. The final test in this group, the **erythrocyte sedimentation rate (ESR),** is a measure of the rate at which red blood cells fall in a column over a one hour period of time. The ESR is often raised in the presence of inflammation and/or infection.

The physician who obtains these tests is looking for evidence of active IBD. When there is anemia, a raised erythrocyte sedimentation rate, an elevated white blood cell count with a "left shift," and an increased platelet count, the physician knows that active inflammation is present. These particular tests, therefore, may be repeated at suitable intervals, first to assist in the recognition of IBD and later in the course of illness to determine whether the inflammation is under control.

Coagulation tests provide information about the patient's ability to clot blood and to control bleeding from the bowel lining. **Prothrombin** is a protein synthesized in the liver. Its formation depends upon the availability of vitamin K and on the liver's ability to synthesize protein. When there is impaired intestinal absorption of vitamin K and/or poor nutrition, the prothrombin time measured in seconds becomes prolonged.

Tests Commonly Performed in IBD

BLOOD AND URINE TESTS

1. Complete blood count (CBC)
2. Platelet count
3. Erythrocyte sedimentation rate (ESR)
4. Coagulation studies (prothrombin time, PTT)
5. Blood chemistries
6. Schilling Test
7. Tests for amebiasis
8. Urinalysis and/or urine culture

STOOL EXAMINATIONS

1. Occult blood
2. Inflammatory cells
3. Culture and sensitivity (C&S)
4. Ova and parasites
5. Toxin assays

RADIOLOGIC PROCEDURES

1. Barium enema examination (BE)
2. Upper GI and small bowel follow-through examination
3. Abdominal ultrasound
4. Abdominal C-T scan
5. Intravenous pyelogram (IVP)

ENDOSCOPIC PROCEDURES

1. Sigmoidoscopy (with biopsy)
2. Colonoscopy (with biopsy)
3. Upper gastrointestinal endoscopy (with biopsy)

Blood chemistries provide important information about nutritional status and general health (total protein, albumin, calcium, phosphorous, magnesium, cholesterol), liver function (bilirubin, alkaline phosphatase, SGOT, SGPT, LDH), kidney function (blood urea nitrogen, creatinine, uric acid) and electrolytes (sodium, potassium, chloride, and bicarbonate). These tests, usually referred to as sequential multiple analysis (SMA-12, SMA-25, etc.), are performed by automatic laboratory equipment, and require only a single tube of blood.

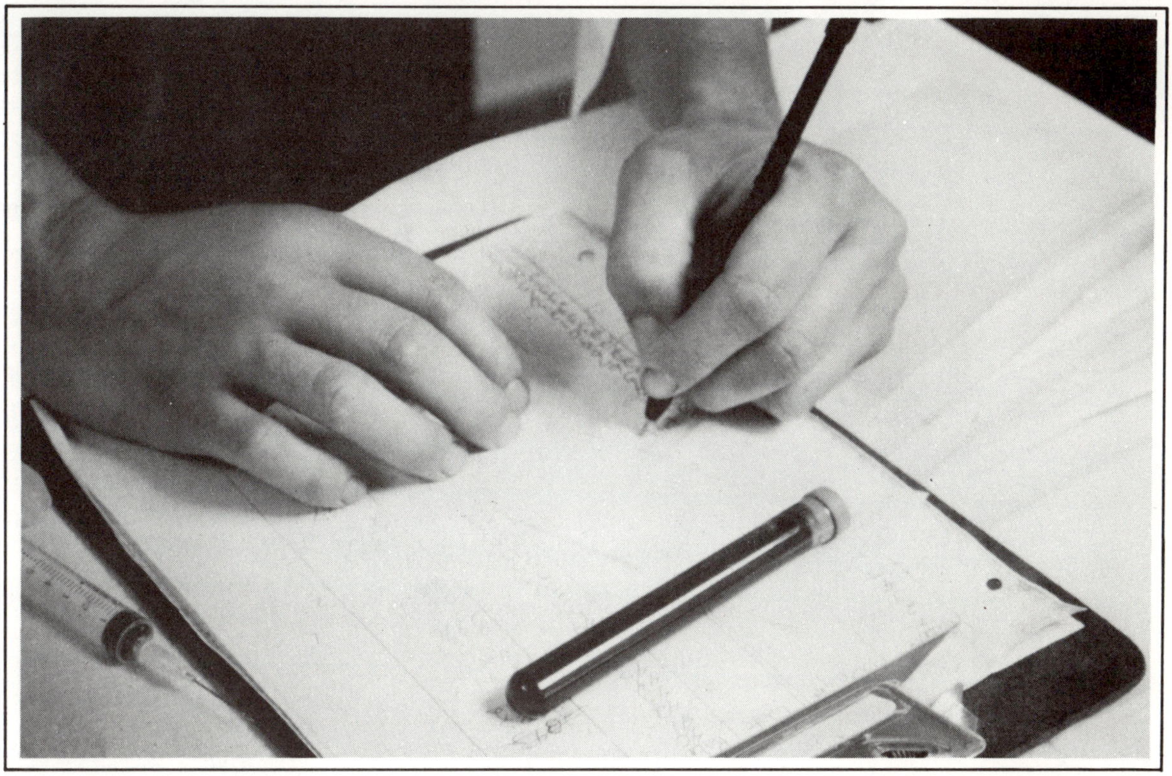

When inflammation involves several feet of lower small intestine or when the terminal ileum has been surgically removed, the absorption of vitamin B-12 may be impaired. After a few years, a vitamin B-12 deficiency may develop resulting in anemia. Absorption of this vitamin can be assessed utilizing the **Schilling test** which measures the excretion into the urine of an orally administered radio-labeled vitamin B-12 preparation. A low urinary excretion rate over a 24-hour period may indicate the need for monthly injections of a vitamin B-12 preparation. A low serum level of vitamin B-12 usually suggests the same conclusion.

Amebiasis is an infection of the colon caused by the parasite, *Entameba histolytica*. It is acquired usually by eating or drinking contaminated food or water. In its severest form, amebiasis causes an inflammation which resembles ulcerative colitis. Occasionally, amebiasis and ulcerative colitis may coexist. Diagnosis depends on identifying the parasite in the stool or in colonic tissue obtained by biopsy. Certain types of blood tests, i.e. indirect hemagglutination antibody (IHA) and complement fixation (CF), provide evidence for active or past infection by the parasite. Since a person with known IBD may acquire an amebic infection, this possibility is kept in mind in evaluating an apparent relapse of IBD.

A **urinalysis** is performed to look for organisms (bacteria), white blood cells, and red blood cells. The finding of bacteria and white cells in large quantities suggests an infection of the urinary tract which may complicate inflammatory bowel disease. Red blood cells in the urine may indicate kidney or bladder stones. A urine culture, sensitivity, and colony count inform the physician whether an infection requires therapy and if so which antibiotic to use.

Stool Examinations

When a person has an acute illness marked by fever, diarrhea, loss of appetite, abdominal cramps, and sometimes nausea and/or vomiting, the physician must exclude an active infection before establishing a diagnosis of inflammatory bowel disease. This requires that the stool be examined.

The physician obtains stool by rectal examination with the gloved finger, the sigmoidoscope, or when the patient provides a sample in a special container. Laxatives or enemas should not be taken prior to the collection of a stool sample in order to avoid irritating the lining of the bowel, destroying certain parasites, or diluting white blood cells.

First, the physician checks for the presence of **occult blood** (hidden blood) by spreading a small portion of stool on specialized paper and adding reagents. The presence of **inflammatory cells** (particularly white blood cells) can be checked by preparing a glass slide with a small portion of stool and examining it with a microscope. A portion of the stool should be sent to the bacteriology lab with a request to determine whether a pathogen (disease-causing organism) such as shigella, salmonella, campylobacter, or yersinia are present **(culture and sensitivity)**. A portion of stool should also be examined as soon as it is obtained for the presence of **ova** (eggs) **and parasites.** Finally, it may be important to send a specimen of stool to a specialized laboratory that can determine whether a **toxin** (poison) produced by clostridia organisms is present. Individuals who may harbor clostridia organisms are those who have received antibiotics which permit the growth of clostridia. The toxin can be responsible for diarrhea and a characteristic inflammation of the lining of the colon. This type of inflammation, unrelated to IBD, can usually be treated successfully with specific antibiotics.

Radiologic Procedures

The **barium enema** examination is used to diagnose or exclude colonic IBD, to determine its status, or to determine whether complications such as strictures have developed. The barium enema examination can also determine whether there is disease of the terminal ileum as it enters the colon through the ileocecal valve. Barium is used alone or combined with air to outline the mucosal lining. In 90 percent of cases, the radiologist can differentiate ulcerative colitis from Crohn's disease based upon the presence or absence of certain radiologic features. A definitive diagnosis is not always possible, and colonoscopic examination may be needed to help in the distinction.

Upper GI and small bowel follow-through examination is performed when the physician wishes to determine if there is inflammation or ulceration of the esophagus, stomach, duodenum, or small intestine. This study helps in establishing a diagnosis of Crohn's desease. When obstruction of the small intestine is suspected, plain x-ray films of the abdomen are undertaken without the use of barium or any other contrast material. Additional films may be taken over a period of time to assess the improvement of obstruction.

It is possible to examine many organs within the abdomen and pelvis using the technique of **diagnostic ultrasound** (sonography). Sound waves pass through the abdomen, encounter structures varying in wall thickness and fluid content, and bounce back to a recording device which visualizes the pattern of sound waves. This technique is considered "non-invasive" since it does not require the use of contrast material by mouth or vein. An additional advantage is that there is no radiation exposure at all. Ultrasound can detect the presence of gallstones and abscesses (collections of pus), both of which can complicate Crohn's disease. A skilled ultrasonographer can differentiate a collection of pus from a swelling of an inflamed loop of intestine. It is even possible for the radiologist to direct a needle into the abscess and to drain it successfully without the need for surgery. Ultrasound can also be used to determine whether the inflamed terminal ileum is obstructing the right ureter causing swelling of the kidney, or whether there is pressure exerted on the urinary bladder.

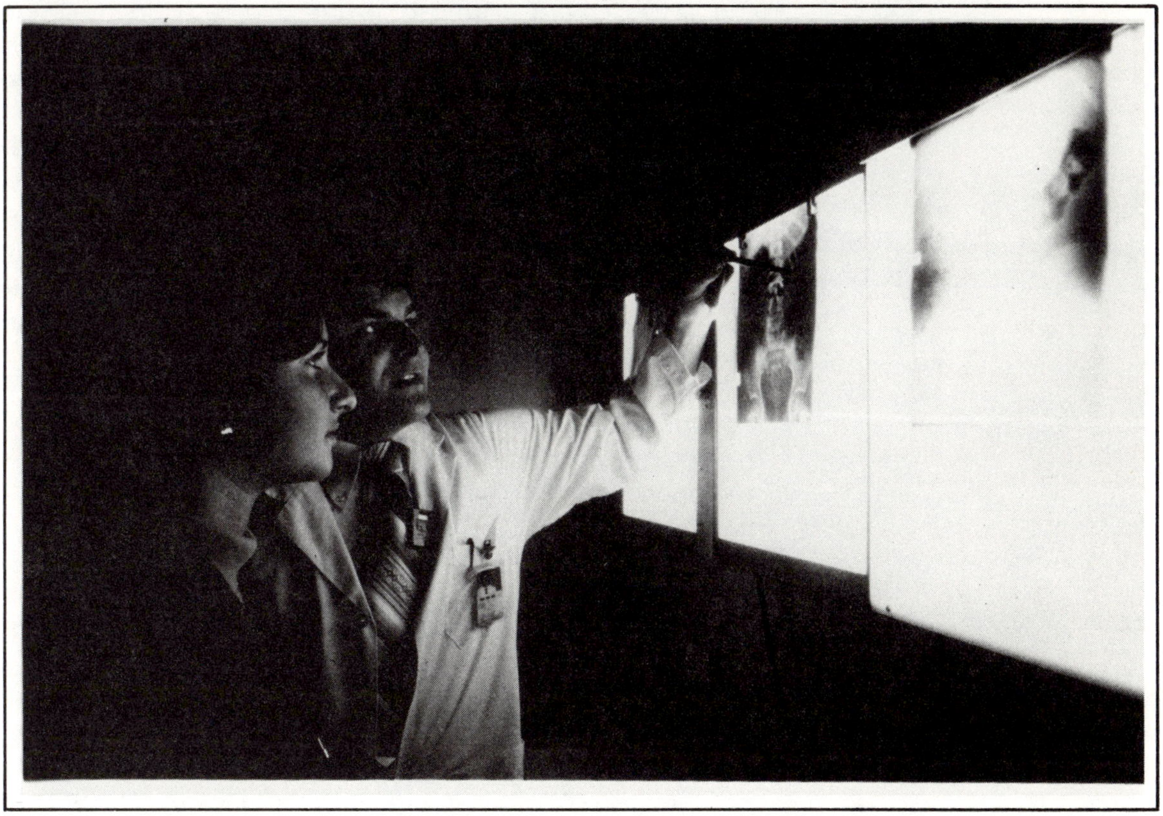

Abdominal C-T scans (computerized tomography) are also used to evaluate organs within the abdomen and pelvic regions. This technique is performed in a special radiology unit housing a large machine capable of examining abdominal and pelvic structures and assembling multiple views of the same structure into three-dimensional configurations. This technique is often complementary to ultrasound examination, although it may also be used independently. Intravenously or orally-administered contrast media are required to evaluate the liver/kidney and bowel loops. It is particularly important to evaluate bowel loops in inflammatory bowel disease when abscess formation is suspected. C-T can also be utilized to guide needles and catheters to facilitate drainage of purulent material from abscess cavities.

The examination of kidneys, ureters, and bladder may be necessary in order to exclude inflammation or obstruction of the urinary tract. Your physician may refer you to a urologist to assist in the evaluation of urinary complaints. The urologist will probably order an **intravenous pyelogram** (IVP) examination. This procedure requires the intravenous administration of an iodine-containing contrast medium which is excreted into the kidneys, ureters, and bladder and outlined on x-rays taken at regular intervals.

Endoscopic Procedures

Endoscopy means looking at the inside of the bowel. The most common endoscopic procedure performed for the evaluation of inflammatory bowel disease is the **sigmoidoscopy.** A rigid or flexible sigmoidoscope is used to examine the rectum and lower sigmoid colon. The entire sigmoid and left colon may be visualized with the flexible instrument, which is longer than the rigid type. In ulcerative colitis, the rectum is almost always involved and the diagnosis can be suspected strongly on sigmoidoscopic examination. When Crohn's disease is suspected, more of the lower left bowel must be examined since the rectum is not always inflamed. The physician may also perform a biopsy of the lining of the bowel, assuming that you have previously provided the required permission and that your coagulation studies are acceptable. Biopsies do not hurt and prolong the procedure only slightly. The mucosal specimens are examined under the microscope to determine whether inflammation is present and how severe it is. This information assists the physician in selecting the proper treatment.

Colonoscopy is endoscopy of the entire colon performed with a flexible instrument 150 cm in length. This procedure is undertaken for a variety of reasons. One is to determine whether IBD is present in any area of the colon or how much of the colon is inflamed. Another is to visualize an abnormality discovered by x-ray examination that is not within the reach of the sigmoidoscope. A third is to help exclude the presence of cancer in a patient with long-standing IBD. Biopsies are frequently obtained during colonscopy, and multiple biopsies are necessary when the purpose of the colonscopy is cancer surveillance.

The esophagus, stomach, duodenum, and first part of the small intestine may be examined with a flexible endoscope 80 cm in length. Endoscopic instruments are now available which allow the examination of a considerable length of upper small intestine **(enteroscopy)**. These procedures may be undertaken if an upper G.I. series suggests inflammation and/or ulceration. Again, biopsies may be necessary to exclude Crohn's disease or fungal infection of the esophagus, which sometimes complicates chronic steroid therapy.

Preparing for Diagnostic Tests

Of the many rights a patient has, one of the most important is the right to receive accurate, complete information about medical tests and examinations. Many factors enter into an individual's acceptance and understanding of the information provided. Age, physical and mental capabilities, language difficulties, level of education and attitude are some of the factors which influence ability to understand. While it is the physician's or nurse's responsibility to recognize any limitations, it is equally important that the patient accept responsibility for understanding the tests and asking pertinent questions.

Editors' Note:

When you are asked to undergo an x-ray or endoscopic procedure, you should always ask the physician what he or she expects to learn from the test, and how that information might alter the management of your IBD. Frequent x-rays are *not* advisable, and if your physician orders them it is not unreasonable for you to ask if the x-ray is essential and why. Physicians are usually very sensitive to the dangers of overexposure to x-rays and should be able to explain the reasons for performing the test. Likewise, barium x-rays and colonoscopies should not be performed if IBD is very active, since this may actually worsen the inflammation.

Bowel Preps

In order for the doctor to have a clear view of the colon during colonoscopy or a barium enema, the colon must be completely free of stool. Therefore, you must carefully and accurately follow special instructions regarding diet, laxatives and enemas.

To begin emptying the bowel, you must stop the ingestion of all solid food. You will probably be asked to drink only clear liquid for a day or two before the examination. Clear liquid includes tea, clear broth, clear gelatin desserts, apple juice, cranberry juice, soda, and water. Clear liquids are those that you can see through and that have no pulp or sediment. (See Chapter 10 for a complete description of the clear liquid diet.)

Diet instructions will probably include fasting from midnight before the examination. When your instructions include nothing to eat or drink (NPO) from midnight, this means that nothing is to be swallowed, not even a drink of water. You may brush your teeth or rinse your mouth, but don't swallow any liquid unless medications must be taken.

Laxatives may be prescribed before your test. These can be made more palatable by mixing them with fruit juice or coke syrup and by drinking the mixture quickly before it separates. There is also a flavored emulsified castor oil which does not separate and is more palatable. If you are experiencing severe diarrhea, abdominal tenderness, or cramps, remind your physician about these symptoms and suggest that strong laxatives be omitted.

The bowel prep for a barium enema will very likely include enemas. Using proper technique when taking or giving an enema is vitally important to obtaining a clean bowel. It is best to lie on the left side because this position uses normal bowel configuration and gravity to assist in the passage of enema fluid through the rectum and into the left side of the colon. Gently insert the tip of the lubricated enema tube through the anus and direct it slowly toward the navel for about 1 1/2 inches. Then redirect the tube so it is pointing toward the base of the spine, and cautiously insert it a few more inches. This technique follows the normal contours of the rectum and will avoid injury to the rectal lining. Hold the enema bag just above the right hip and allow the contents to flow slowly up into the colon. If the fluid is allowed to run in too rapidly, it may stimulate the rectum to expel the fluid prematurely. Elevating the buttocks on a pillow may help in retaining more of the fluid.

Planning ahead reduces the anxiety and stress associated with an unfamiliar experience.

Some physicians may prefer that you use a different type of bowel preparation. Instead of taking laxatives and enemas, you may be asked to drink a special liquid which will cause diarrhea and thus cleanse the bowel. This preparation requires you to drink a glass of the solution every 15 minutes for 4 hours. It is important to follow the directions exactly. You may feel bloated drinking this much liquid, but this feeling will lessen as you empty your bowel.

You should always be sure to have access to a bathroom before you begin the prep. If you are to take enemas on the morning of the test, be sure to allow enough extra time to expel the enemas and still arrive on time. It is also important to collect all the equipment you will need and make sure you understand the instructions prior to the day of the procedure. Planning ahead reduces the anxiety and stress associated with an unfamiliar experience.

Sigmoidoscopy

Preparation for this examination usually includes one or two enemas within an hour or two prior to the procedure. If you are having a flexible sigmoidoscopy, you may be instructed either to fast or to take only liquids for 4 to 6 hours before the examination. For rigid sigmoidoscopy, there are usually no dietary restrictions. You may take your daily medications unless instructed otherwise by the doctor. You usually will not be given any medications prior to the test so you will be able to drive yourself home.

You will be asked to lie on a table on your left side with your knees flexed, or on a special table which can be adjusted so you will be lying in a knee-chest or jacknife position. Your body will be draped with a sheet so that only your buttocks are exposed for the examination.

The doctor will first examine your rectum with a gloved finger. He will then insert the sigmoidoscope, which may give you a mild sensation of wanting to move your bowels. You may feel some cramping or gas discomfort during the examination, especially if the doctor injects small amounts of air to help visualize the lining. You may notice some abdominal pressure as the sigmoidoscope is advanced through the lower bowel. These feelings should be completely tolerable and not painful. Sometimes a biopsy (tiny bit of tissue) may be removed for microscopic examination. You will not feel any discomfort when the biopsy is taken. The procedure itself takes about 5 to 10 minutes.

During the examination, try to let your abdominal muscles relax in order to prevent discomfort caused by muscle tension. Try to breathe rhythmically. Some air may remain in the bowel after the instrument is removed. You will feel more comfortable if you expel this air. A bathroom should be readily available to you.

Colonoscopy

When preparing for a colonoscopy, it is advisable to discontinue aspirin products, bulking agents, and iron preparations for about a week before the examination. Aspirin increases the risk of bleeding if biopsies are required, bulking agents make cleansing of the bowel more difficult, and iron preparations blacken the stool. Do not take any medications from midnight before the examination unless advised to do so by your physician.

Prior to colonoscopy, you will be asked to sign a consent form after the doctor has explained the procedure and answered all your questions. Be sure to let the doctor or nurse know if you are allergic to any drugs or adhesive tape. You will be asked to remove any dentures or contact lenses. Medications will be given by needle into your vein or your muscle and will begin to make you feel sleepy and relaxed. You will then be asked to turn on your left side and the room will be darkened.

The doctor will examine your rectum with a gloved finger and then insert the flexible colonoscope tube gently into your rectum. He/she will advance the tube slowly through your colon, examining the lining thoroughly. You may feel some abdominal cramping from the air which the doctor injects into your colon. You may also be asked to change position to help with passage of the colonoscope. Fluoroscopy (x-ray) equipment may be used to evaluate the location of the instrument. Occasionally during the examination, the nurse may apply pressure with her hand to your abdomen to help with the passage of the instrument. Biopsies may be taken for microscopic examination, but these should not cause you any pain or discomfort.

The colonoscopic examination takes about 20 minutes to one hour. After the procedure, you will be moved to a quiet room to sleep or rest until the effect of the medication partially wears off. You may feel some bloating from the air which remains in the colon. You may feel more comfortable if you expel this air, but it is not advisable to force this.

It is very important that you be escorted home after the examination and that you remain at home until the next day. The reason for this is that the medications that you receive for sedation may have a prolonged effect that would interfere with your ability to drive an automobile or even cross a busy street unescorted.

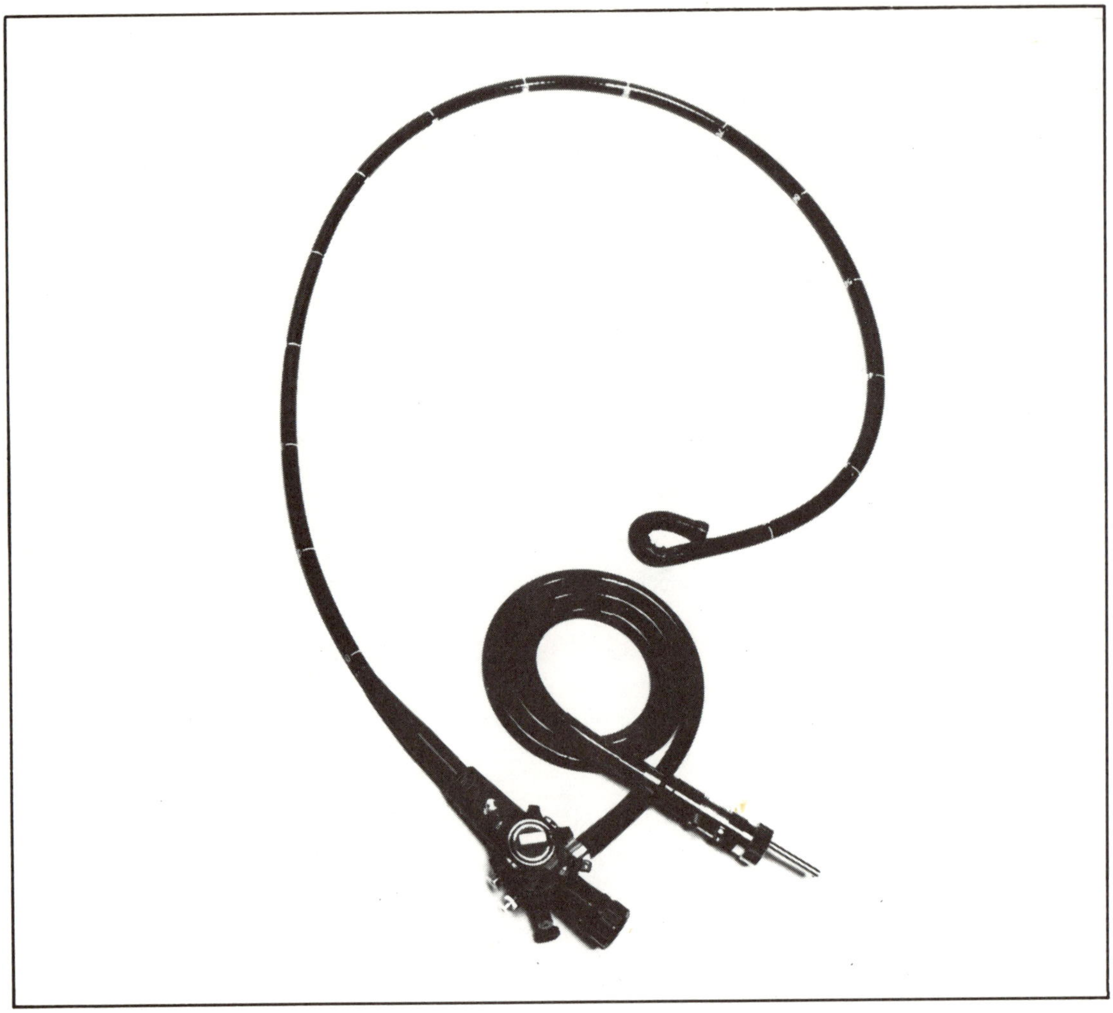

The Fiberoptic Colonoscope

Occasionally, local irritation of the vein occurs at the site of the medication injection. You should use warm soaks to this area if necessary. If you notice excessive pain, redness, or warmth at the injection site, be sure to notify your physician. You should also report any fever, abdominal pain or rectal bleeding. If a biopsy was perfomed, aspirin products should be avoided for a few days.

Upper Gastrointestinal Endoscopy

In order for the physician to have a clear view of your upper digestive tract, your stomach must be completely empty. It is very important to take nothing to eat or drink from midnight before the examination. This includes lozenges, hard candy and antacids which can coat and discolor the lining of the esophagus and interfere with the accuracy of the examination. You should check with your doctor whether to take your usual medications.

As with a colonoscopy, you will be asked to sign a consent form to authorize the doctor to perform the examination. All dentures and contact lenses and any constricting undergarments must be removed prior to the start of the examination. Medications will be given by injection into your vein or muscle which will make you sleepy and relaxed. The physician may also spray the back of your throat with an anesthetic spray to numb the area and to prevent you from gagging. You will be asked to turn onto your left side and a small plastic mouth piece will be placed between your teeth. You will be able to breathe through your mouth or nose, whichever is more comfortable for you.

When you are completely relaxed and nearly asleep, the room will be darkened and the physician will help you swallow the flexible endoscope tube. It is normal to feel a gagging sensation, but this will pass. Often a biopsy (tiny bit of tissue) is taken for microscopic examination. You will feel no discomfort when the biopsy is taken. Bloating occurs because air is introduced to enable visualization of the stomach. Belching is common. Throughout the procedure, a nurse will be suctioning saliva from your mouth and throat.

The procedure lasts about 15-30 minutes. After the endoscope is removed, you will be moved to a quiet room to sleep or rest until the effect of the medication partially wears off (usually about 1 hour). Unless the doctor or the nurse instructs you otherwise, you will be able to resume your regular diet about 4 hours after the procedure.

You may notice a slight scratchy throat following the procedure. This can be relieved by lozenges, gargles or by drinking liquids. If this symptom persists over 24 hours or worsens, notify your doctor. Also, be sure to report any fever, chest or abdominal pain, or passage of bloody or black stools. As with the colonoscopy, you must be driven home by someone who will assume responsibility for your safety.

For Further Information...

The X-Ray Information Book, by Priscilla W. Laws and The Public Citizen Health Research Group. New York: Farrar, Straus & Giroux, 1983. (This book may be purchased for $3.25 from The Public Citizen Health Research Group, Dept. 222, 2000 P Street, N.W., Washington, D.C. 20036.)

3

IBD Medications And Their Side Effects

Since there is no medical cure for inflammatory bowel disease, the goals of medical treatment are to suppress the inflammatory response, permit healing of tissue, and relieve the symptoms of diarrhea, abdominal pain, and fever. As inflammation subsides and symptoms resolve, the person with IBD enters a quiescent phase of illness called a remission. This remission may last for a few weeks or for many years. At times, the remission is prolonged only if medications are continued; at other times, the remission persists even after medications have been discontinued. A remission does not necessarily mean that all active inflammation has subsided or that the inflamed tissue has healed completely. A remission *does* mean that the person is once again comfortable and able to resume normal activities.

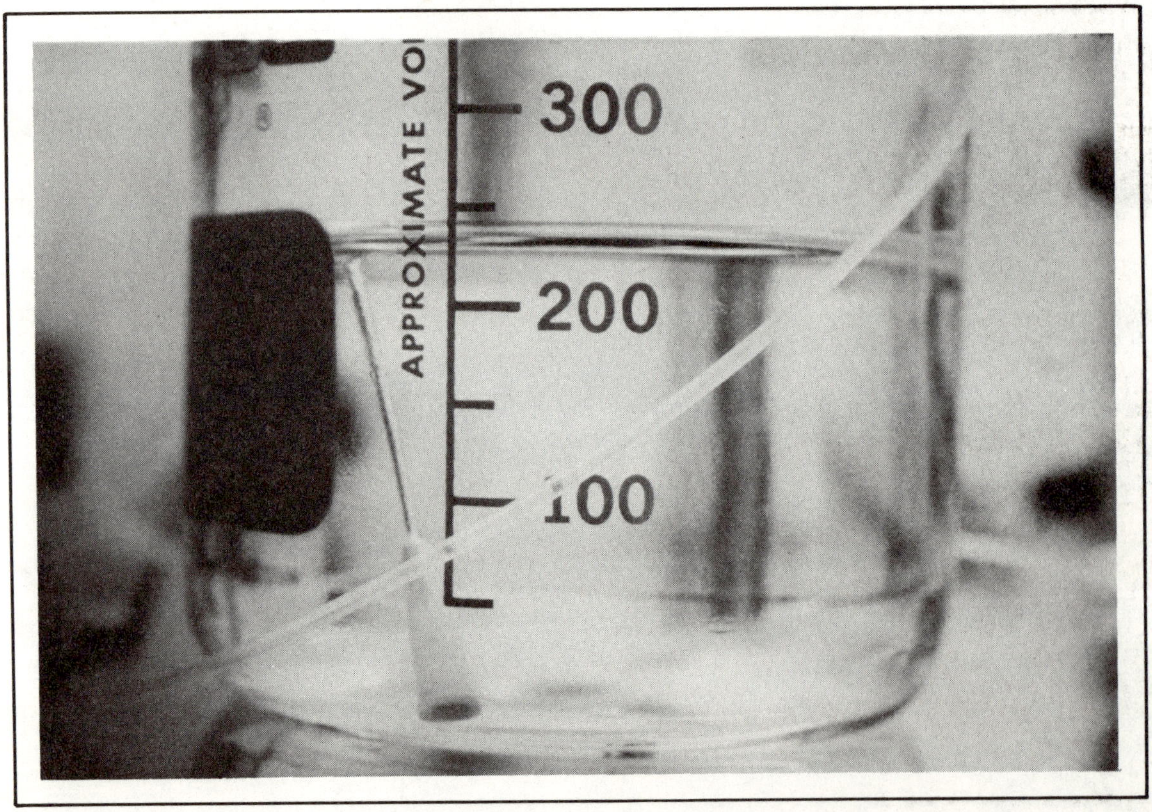

For each of the major medications used to treat IBD, we have provided information about its use, its doses and available preparations, and commonly encountered side effects. This chapter concludes with a discussion of the problem of addiction caused by the use of drugs to control pain and diarrhea.

Sulfasalazine: Its Use in IBD

Sulfasalazine is an effective treatment for mild to moderate episodes of ulcerative colitis. In severe episodes, the disease either does not respond adequately to sulfasalazine or the response is not rapid enough. (Severe ulcerative colitis usually requires a corticosteroid preparation administered intravenously.) After ulcerative colitis has responded to sulfasalazine, the drug is usually continued in order to prolong the clinical remission. This recommendation is based on evidence that although people with ulcerative colitis can have flare-ups while taking sulfasalazine, the risk is significantly lower if the drug is continued.

Sulfasalazine is also effective in treating Crohn's disease which is either confined entirely to the colon or involves both the ileum and colon. Available data suggest that this medication is much less helpful in treating Crohn's disease confined to the ileum (ileitis). Nevertheless, many physicians begin treating ileitis patients with sulfasalazine rather than the more powerful corticosteroid agents, on the chance that it might help. Unlike its usefulness in ulcerative colitis, sulfasalazine does not help maintain a remission in Crohn's disease. Also, taking maintenance doses of sulfasalazine does *not* prevent recurrences of Crohn's disease after surgical removal of diseased tissue.

Preparations and Doses

Sulfasalazine is available as an oral preparation in several forms: a tablet; an enteric coated tablet that helps prevent upper digestive symptoms; and a suspension for people who may have difficulty swallowing a large tablet. The usual dosage is 2 to 4 grams a day (4-8 tablets). For some people, a dose of 2 grams provides excellent therapy, and there is then no need to increase the dose further. Taking sulfasalazine with meals or with a snack helps prevent digestive side effects which sometimes develop with this medication.

Sulfasalazine contains two active ingredients: a sulfa preparation (sulfapyridine) and an aspirin-like drug (5-aminosalicylic acid or 5-ASA). Most of the drug reaches the colon intact when bacterial enzymes break the bond that links the two ingredients. The sulfapyridine is absorbed into the bloodstream and is responsible for almost all of the unpleasant and, at times, serious side effects, while providing few, if any, therapeutic benefits. The 5-ASA is absorbed only minimally into the bloodstream and is the ingredient that suppresses tissue inflammation by acting on the colon (topically) before being eliminated in the stool.

You may be wondering why it is not possible simply to take 5-ASA *without* the sulfapyridine. The reason is that the 5-ASA molecule (without its sulfapyridine carrier molecule) is absorbed quickly in the upper small intestine and excreted in the urine before it can reach the colon where it has its beneficial effect. Currently, a variety of oral forms are being developed which circumvent this absorption problem. One preparation links two 5-ASA molecules. Another links 5—ASA to an inert compound which "delivers" it to the colon. A third uses an acrylic-based resin to coat 5-ASA so that it is not released until it reaches the less acid environment of the colon. In addition, enema and suppository forms of 5-ASA which do not have a "delivery" problem will be available shortly.

Studies in Europe, where various forms of 5-ASA are already in use, have shown that 5-ASA is effective in suppressing inflammation in both ulcerative colitis and Crohn's disease without serious side effects (although few long-term studies are available).

Side Effects of Sulfasalazine

The most serious side effect caused by sulfasalazine involves the bone marrow, where blood elements are manufactured. The physician can monitor the effects of sulfasalazine on the bone marrow by measuring the concentration of white blood cells, red blood cells, and platelets in blood. Sulfasalazine may suppress the synthesis of all three of these blood cell types in the bone marrow. You should know that bone marrow toxicity caused by sulfasalazine occurs very rarely and can be discovered quickly with one simple blood test—the complete blood count (CBC). A CBC should be obtained at some regular interval during the first few months of treatment and then at some periodic interval thereafter. If bone marrow depression is found, you will be instructed not to take sulfasalazine or any other medications containing sulfa.

A second serious side effect involves red blood cells after they have been manufactured by the bone marrow. In some people, red blood cells react to the presence of sulfa by undergoing a premature breakdown called hemolysis. Periodic measurement of complete blood count alerts the physician to this problem. Other potentially serious side effects include acute pancreatitis, hepatitis, and pneumonitis. Fortunately, all of these side effects are extremely rare.

There are other side effects that are distressing but not serious. These include headache, nausea, vomiting, and loss of appetite. Sometimes, when sulfasalazine therapy is begun with smaller than usual doses, these side effects can be eliminated. For example, therapy can begin with a dose of one tablet of sulfasalazine twice daily for two or three days, and gradually increase to higher doses.

Fever and rash are side effects which indicate an allergic reaction to sulfasalazine. It was once thought that these symptoms precluded any additional attempt at treatment with sulfasalazine. Experience has now shown that fever and/or rash can often be prevented if the medication is restarted in extremely small doses. This process is called desensitization. Initial doses can be as small as one-quarter of a tablet daily for several days, increasing to one-quarter of a tablet twice daily for several days, and slowly increasing to larger amounts. Complete blood counts and platelet counts are advisable at some periodic interval during this process. If fever or rash recurs during this gradual process, further therapy with sulfasalazine should be abandoned.

Editors' Note

If your physician orders blood tests to monitor possible toxicity of sulfasalazine, you should obtain these tests on schedule and check with your physician to make sure that the test results have been received. You must not assume that laboratory results are always received by the physician and that the physician would have called the patient if a problem exists. Check with your physician to be absolutely sure that the laboratory reports have been received and interpreted and that it is safe to continue treatment with sulfasalazine.

Corticosteroids in IBD

Corticosteroids are effective in the treatment of both Crohn's disease and ulcerative colitis. These drugs reduce tissue inflammation and thereby relieve symptoms such as diarrhea, rectal bleeding, abdominal pain, and fever. These drugs also relieve other "systemic" symptoms associated with IBD, including joint pains, and inflammation of the skin and eyes. After ulcerative colitis has been brought under control, maintenance therapy with low-dose corticosteroids *does not* prevent a flare-up. (You will recall that maintenance therapy with sulfasalazine *can* prevent a flare-up in ulcerative colitis.) In Crohn's disease, maintenance therapy with corticosteroids does not prevent a flare-up, nor does it prevent a recurrence of the disease after surgery.

At times in both ulcerative colitis and in Crohn's disease, corticosteroids and sulfasalazine are administered simultaneously. However, it is not known whether this combination is more beneficial than a corticosteroid agent administered by itself.

Preparations and Doses

Corticosteroids can be administered in many forms. Oral preparations include prednisone and methylprednisolone (Medrol) tablets. The drug can also be given by intravenous or intramuscular injection in the form of hydrocortisone or methylprednisolone (Solu-Medrol), and by rectal instillation as an enema or foam. Intravenous or intramuscular steroids are needed when patients are unable to take oral medication or are acutely ill and require a prompt therapeutic response. Corticosteroid enemas and foams are helpful in healing active inflammation of rectum and/or sigmoid colon.

A related medication sometimes used in IBD is corticotropin (ACTH). ACTH is a hormone secreted by the pituitary gland to stimulate the release of cortisol, the body's own form of corticosteroid, from the adrenal gland. ACTH is available only as an intramuscular or intravenous preparation, and is considered as effective as corticosteroids in reducing tissue inflammation. Some physicians feel that in some situations it may be even more effective, and may prevent suppression of the adrenal gland sometimes caused by synthetic corticosteroids.

Corticosteroid enemas, foams and suppositories are especially helpful in relieving uncomfortable rectal symptoms, particularly tenesmus, the repetitive urge to move the bowels. Tenesmus is triggered by rectal inflammation and is relieved only temporarily by the evacuation of a small amount of liquid rectal contents. Steroid preparations inserted or injected into the rectum reduce inflammation and promote healing in two ways. They act topically (on the bowel surface) and are partially absorbed, delivering a systemic effect. These preparations are helpful in ulcerative proctitis, ulcerative colitis and in Crohn's disease affecting the rectum and sigmoid colon.

Corticosteroids available for rectal use include suppositories, rectal foam, and enemas. A suppository such as Anusol-HC, which contains 10 mg of hydrocortisone, is easy to insert and may be effective for mild proctitis. Rectal preparations that include corticosteroids as a foam include Cortifoam, which contains 80 mg of hydrocortisone with each application, and Proctofoam-HC, which contains 5 mg of hydrocortisone with each application. Foam preparations come with an applicator which eases their insertion into the rectum. Since these foams contain mostly air, they do not cause the urge to evacuate and can be easily retained.

When active inflammation extends well into the sigmoid colon, foams may not be dispersed deep enough to coat this tissue, and enemas may be needed. The most familiar of these products is Cortenema, which contains 100 mg of hydrocortisone in a 60 ml container. You are instructed to insert the exposed tip of the plastic container and gently squeeze the container to force fluid into the rectum. By trial and error, each person can determine how firmly and rapidly to squeeze the container to permit the delivery of the fluid into the rectum without stimulating the urge to evacuate. Another enema preparation is called Medrol-Enpak. This kit contains an enema bag, plastic tubing, and vials of Medrol powder each containing 40 mg of Medrol. One advantage of Medrol-Enpak is that the volume of fluid used to dilute the powder can be individualized. The starting volume of fluid (90 ml) can be increased gradually to the full capacity of the enema bag (180 ml) to deliver the medication high in the sigmoid colon and even into the descending colon.

Rectal steroids are usually self-administered at bedtime in the hope that the patient will retain them through the night. They can also be administered in the morning if symptoms are severe enough to require therapy twice daily. It is important to bear in mind that people taking rectal steroids absorb a portion of this medication and are therefore at risk of developing some of the same side effects as those who receive steroids by another route.

A new steroid enema, tixocortal pivalate, is now being developed. In clinical studies, this preparation appears to promote rapid healing of inflamed rectal tissue with virtually no systemic cortisone activity.

Side Effects of Corticosteroids

Serious side effects caused by corticosteroid therapy do not occur often but are a cause for concern when they do occur. These include thinning of the bones (osteoporosis), elevated blood sugar, hypertension, cataracts, increased susceptibility to infection, and serious personality changes. There are other side effects that are less serious but at times troublesome, including loss of hair, acne, rounding of the face, fluid retention, and stretch marks over the abdomen. The potential for side effects diminishes as the dose of corticosteroids is reduced and usually disappears completely when the medication is discontinued. Experience has also shown that when corticosteroids are administered every other day, the potential for serious side effects is minimized. This method of treatment has been particularly helpful with adolescents who are often greatly troubled by the side effects of steroids. Alternate day therapy may not be feasible if the disease process is very active.

Another possible side effect of corticosteroid therapy is adrenal insufficiency. Our adrenal glands normally manufacture small amounts of a corticosteroid hormone which helps in responding to any "stress" on the body, such as infection or surgery. When synthetic steroids are given as medication, the body's production of its own steroids temporarily shuts down. The aim of all steroid therapy is to gradually decrease the dose so that the adrenal gland can begin working again. In some individuals this may take some time, and the adrenal gland may not function normally for up to a full year after therapy has been stopped. People with adrenal insufficiency may require an additional "boost" of corticosteroids if they develop infections or need surgery.

Immunosuppressive Agents in IBD

Immunosuppressives are substances which alter the body's normal immune response to disease or to antigens (foreign substances within the body). They have been used in the treatment of the so-called autoimmune diseases–diseases in which the tissues are attacked by the body's own antibodies–and in preventing the rejection of transplanted organs. Immunosuppressive agents, such as azathioprine (Imuran) and 6-mercaptopurine (6-MP) have a limited role in the treatment of ulcerative colitis. This is because sulfasalazine and corticosteroid agents are usually quite effective, and because physicians are concerned about potential side effects of this group of medications (see below). For these reasons, immunosuppressive agents are not generally used as single agents in the treatment of ulcerative colitis. Some physicians prescribe immunosuppressive agents when ulcerative colitis requires large doses of corticosteroids on a long term basis for control of symptoms. In this case, the immunosuppressive drug may permit a gradual reduction in the dose of steroids and reduce the possibility of side effects caused by continuous high dose steroid therapy.

Immunosuppressive drugs may permit a gradual reduction in the dose of steroids and reduce the possibility of side effects caused by continuous high dose steroid therapy.

In Crohn's disease, immunosuppressive agents are often administered together with sulfasalazine and/or corticosteroids. Using immunosuppressives in this way often results in general improvement of symptoms and in the closure of fistulas. In one study, fistulas closed completely in approximately 40 percent of patients and showed significant improvement in an additional 25 percent. After improvement has taken place, the dose of corticosteroids can be reduced and at times discontinued completely while the patient continues to receive an immunosuppressive drug. Immunosuppressive agents may take as long as four months to achieve results. For this reason sulfasalazine and/or corticosteroids are usually continued during this period. Once immunosuppressive therapy is discontinued, relapses may occur, but these often respond to reintroduction of the medication.

Preparations and Doses

The usual oral dose of 6-mercaptopurine (6-MP) is 1.5 mg per kilogram of body weight per day. The usual dose of azathioprine is 1.5-2.0 mg per kilogram. If you are taking immunosuppressives, it is important to maintain a very close communication with your physician to prevent the development of serious side effects (see below). Blood tests must be obtained at regular intervals, including a complete blood count and platelet count. You must not assume that the physician receives a report of each blood test and that it is safe to continue this medication. It is your responsibility to receive a verbal communication either from the physician or one of his staff that the results of tests permit you to continue with this medication.

Side Effects of Immunosuppressives

Immunosuppressive agents may cause depressed production of certain blood cells—namely white blood cells and platelets—in the bone marrow. An abnormally low white blood count may permit a serious infection to develop. A reduced platelet count may cause bleeding. Fortunately, a routine, periodic complete blood count and platelet count provides sufficient warning to the physician that the medication dose should be reduced or discontinued altogether. Other side effects that occur very rarely include nausea, fever, rash, pancreatitis, and hepatitis. There has been no evidence of increased cancer incidence among patients with IBD who have received immunosuppressive agents for intervals up to 5 to 10 years, although large numbers of patients remain to be studied.

Despite many reported successes, immunosuppressive therapy has not yet gained widespread use. Additional favorable experience may convince other physicians that these agents are safe, effective, and helpful in specific situations where other therapy has not been successful.

Antibiotics: Metronidazole

Metronidazole is an antibiotic which is used to treat a variety of parasitic and bacterial infections. While its use in ulcerative colitis is untested and uncertain, in Crohn's disease, metronidazole has been successful in treating severe perianal sinus tracts and fistulas as well as the general symptoms of Crohn's colitis. Metronidazole is probably beneficial because of its antibacterial activity, but there may be some immunologic properties of this medication as well.

The dose, usually administered orally, is 15 to 20 mg per kilogram of body weight per day. A favorable response may not take place for several weeks. If symptoms return when metronidazole is reduced or discontinued, restarting the medication usually brings relief.

One important side effect occurring at high doses is numbness of the lower legs and feet. In most instances, these symptoms disappear when the dose is lowered or the medication is discontinued. In rare instances, these symptoms have persisted indefinitely. Other side effects include nausea, a metallic taste in the mouth, discoloration of the urine, and loss of appetite. As with many medications, there is always a concern about possible long-term side effects, including the development of cancer. Serious long term side effects of metronidazole have not been identified, although further study is required.

Other Antibiotics

Antibiotics are best used to treat the infections that often complicate ulcerative colitis or Crohn's disease. Once the lining of the small or large intestine is damaged, bacteria may penetrate the bowel wall and cause either a local or systemic infection. When a flare-up of disease is associated with a high fever and other signs of infection, an antibiotic or combination of antibiotics should be administered intravenously. Because steroids may mask important signs of infection such as fever, antibiotics are often used during the first 7 to 10 days of therapy with corticosteroid agents.

Among several side effects that may occur with antibiotic therapy, one that is easily recognized is a secondary yeast infection of the mouth and throat (thrush). This infection is caused by *Candida albicans* and occurs more often in people who are quite ill and are receiving multiple medications including antibiotics and/or steroids. Whitish plaques appear on the lining of the cheeks, tongue, or throat, and there may also be a sore throat or pain in the upper chest on swallowing, meaning that the infection has spread to the esophagus. If you are receiving antibiotics and/or corticosteroids, make it a point to check for these signs. Treatment consists of oral solutions that can be gargled and swallowed several times a day.

Antidiarrheal Agents

Diarrhea is a major symptom in IBD. It is important to reduce the number of loose bowel movements to provide more restful sleep, encourage food intake, and to allow daily activities to continue normally. At the same time, over-use of medications to reduce diarrhea may lead to serious complications. As a general rule, you should be satisfied with modest but distinct improvement in diarrhea rather than strive for the total elimination of the problem.

There are several categories of drugs that help in relieving diarrhea. In IBD, the substances used most often to control diarrhea are narcotics or synthetic narcotics. Examples of these substances are codeine, diphenoxylate (Lomotil), and loperamide (Imodium). Loperamide has an important second property of tightening the anal sphincter and helping to prevent incontinence. A second group of drugs increases the intestinal absorption of fluid and electrolytes. Corticosteroid agents have this property, and improvement in diarrhea with these drugs is probably a reflection of this action more than a reduction in tissue inflammation. Other medications that may help to improve absorption of fluid and electroyltes are cloninide and the phenothiazines. These medications also have important side effects and should be used cautiously.

Cholestyramine (Questran) is another medication that may help to reduce diarrhea when there is either extensive inflammation of the terminal ileum or surgical removal of a portion of the terminal ileum. Cholestyramine is a non-absorbable resin that binds bile salts and other materials in the small intestine. When absorption of bile salts is incomplete (a result of disease or surgical removal of the terminal ileum), unabsorbed bile salts enter the colon and cause it to secrete an excessive amount of fluid and electrolytes. Cholestyramine prevents this diarrhea by binding these bile salts before they reach the colon. One package (4 grams) dissolved in a glass of water before breakfast is usually all that is required to achieve a therapeutic benefit. Additional doses can be administered before lunch and dinner if needed. If diarrhea does not improve and if there is weight loss, cholestyramine should be discontinued.

The most important side effect of narcotics and other agents used to control diarrhea and cramps is the development of toxic megacolon, paralysis of the motor activity of the colon which causes distension and potential perforation. Early symptoms include an increase in abdominal pain, distension, and tenderness, and persistence or increase in fever. There are also fewer bowel movements which ordinarily would be interpreted as a sign of improvement. Toxic megacolon is a potentially very serious condition that requires hospitalization.

Narcotic Dependence in IBD

The use of narcotic substances to control pain and diarrhea creates several serious problems for the person with IBD. First, narcotic use diminishes symptoms without treating the underlying illness. Second, these drugs cause the body to become tolerant and to require larger and larger doses to achieve the same result. Third, narcotic use often creates a separate set of bowel symptoms ("narcotic bowel syndrome") superimposed on IBD, which may become a separate clinical problem, and may necessitate treatment in the hospital.

We do not know how common narcotic dependence is in IBD. In a recent study of 43 IBD patients referred to a psychiatrist, 30 percent were found to be dependent on some form of addicting medication. While this high percentge is probably not typical of all people with IBD, the best estimate is that about one in twenty people will develop some problem of drug dependence in the course of their therapy.

The best way to combat this problem is to have some knowledge about how these drugs can be used safely and to work with a single physician who is also knowledgeable about this. Often, people with IBD have several doctors involved in their care: a family doctor, a gastroenterologist and, at times a surgeon. The most important factor in preventing narcotic dependence is to "appoint" one physician in this team to be the only one to prescribe narcotics. This allows good monitoring of the need for narcotics.

Narcotics commonly used for pain are codeine, meperidine (Demerol) and oxycodone (Percocet and Percodan). For more severe pain and usually only in the hospital, injectable narcotics are used, such as pentazocaine (Talwin), opium alkaloids, and morphine sulfate. These drugs can be used safely without causing drug dependence as long as they are carefully monitored by a physician, the dose gradually reduced, and the medication discontinued when the acute episode resolves. When pain exceeds two to three weeks in duration, narcotics are not a good regular treatment because of the development of tolerance and the risk of drug dependence. In addition, the regular use of narcotics can actually *increase* a person's sensitivity to pain. Persistent pain may indicate a need to change the medical management of IBD.

For diarrhea, the situation is somewhat different. The drugs commonly used are diphenoxylate (Lomotil), deodorized tincture of opium, and codeine. The risk of addiction in still present with these drugs, but it is less than with the other narcotics.

The problem is often that the earliest signs of addiction are known only to the person taking the narcotic, and he or she will often deny them.

The signs of drug dependence should be familiar to all IBD patients and their families. The earliest sign generally is preoccupation with the drug (such as counting the time until the next dose) or use of drug for reasons other than to control pain or diarrhea (for example as a sleeping medication). The next danger signs to watch for are the use of increasing doses or a shortening of the time interval between doses. At this point, withdrawal symptoms (anxiety, cramps, sweating, irritability) may be felt if a dose is missed. These symptoms indicate a physical addiction. If this situation is allowed to progress, the person may seek to obtain more medication (commonly by "losing" prescriptions or consulting other doctors with the intention of obtaining a narcotic). Family members or friends may begin to notice that the person is doing less, "looks spacey," and may have slurred speech. These signs should be discussed with the doctor immediately. The problem is often that the earliest signs of addiction are known only to the person taking the narcotic, and he or she will often deny them. This is unfortunate because if detected early, drug dependence is not yet fully developed and can be more easily treated.

A word should be said about the uses of narcotics in people with IBD who have had a prior drug problem or still do. Such a problem could be the use of cocaine, tranquilizers, alcohol, or even marijuana. At least one in 14 young people have such a problem and some of them develop IBD. It is crucial to let your physician know of this problem, even if drugs have not been a problem for years. If your doctor knows this, he or she can use extra caution in prescribing narcotics.

4

Skin Care In IBD

Skin problems are a particularly troublesome complication of inflammatory bowel disease. In many cases the only skin trouble is acne, which is not caused by IBD but is often made worse by taking corticosteroids. At other times, the skin problem may be a direct manifestation of the underlying *systemic* disease—either Crohn's disease or ulcerative colitis. Mouth sores and erythema nodosum are skin disorders of this type. Other common problems arise in the perianal area, the area immediately surrounding the anus. Each of these IBD-related skin disorders requires special attention and specific treatment. In this chapter, we present explanations of each condition and suggestions which should help make these conditions more tolerable.

Coping with a case of acne makes adjusting to IBD all the more difficult for the young person.

Acne

Because many people with Crohn's disease and ulcerative colitis require corticosteroids at some time in the course of their treatment, the problem of acne may be made worse by these medications. Young people who are already troubled by acne may require corticosteroids which will likely make the acne worse. Coping with a case of acne makes adjusting to IBD all the more difficult for the young person.

Understanding the nature of acne is important in order to help you plan effective treatment. First of all, acne is *not* caused by dirt or pores blocked by dirt. The primary abnormality in acne is blockage of the secretions within the tiny pores of the skin. Corticosteroids seem to aggravate this process. Acne brought on by corticosteroids does not usually cause blackheads (blocked pores) and whiteheads (pores with local infection), but most often causes an unsightly inflammation under the skin in the form of small, uniform red bumps.

A few principles of skin care may be helpful. When acne is present, the skin should be kept clean and free of grease and oil. Washing the face twice a day with a mild soap with no added fragrance, coloring, or chemicals is beneficial. Avoid vigorous rubbing. After the skin is washed and the soap rinsed away, the skin should be dried by patting rather than rubbing. Make-up and skin moisturizers should be oil-free. Avoid using oily hair dressings or hair sprays.

A useful over-the-counter preparation is benzoyl peroxide, which acts against bacteria and tends to clear the pores. Other medications available to counteract acne usually require a prescription. Fortunately, acne usually improves when the corticosteroid medication is decreased or discontinued.

Mouth Sores

A common problem experienced by many people with IBD is aphthous ulcers of the mouth or "canker sores." These sores can be annoying, especially while eating. While there is no specific treatment, mild mouth rinses such as lukewarm, dilute salt water are soothing. Astringent mouth washes should be avoided. Liquid antacid or Kaopectate applied directly to the sore can be soothing. If the sores persist, you should consult your physician. Prescription medications such as topical anesthetics, antibiotic rinses, and some antihistamines are available to reduce inflammation and tenderness. The frequency and severity of mouth sores generally improve as the IBD is brought under control.

Erythema Nodosum and Pyoderma Gangrenosum

These are two rather serious skin conditions that occur specifically with IBD. It is not known exactly how or why these skin conditions arise, but it is comforting to know that they tend to improve as IBD improves.

Since an episode of erythema nodosum may signify an imminent flare-up of IBD, you should always inform your physician if bumps such as these occur.

Erythema nodosum causes red, tender raised bumps to appear, usually on the shins. Elevating the legs as often as possible helps to reduce discomfort. Arranging a holder to keep bedsheets off the legs is also helpful. Since an episode of erythema nodosum may signify an imminent flare-up of IBD, you should *always* inform your physician if bumps such as these occur. Erythema nodosum is usually a temporary (although painful) problem which leaves no permanent marks and improves as IBD is treated.

Pyoderma gangrenosum is a rare skin condition which is somewhat more likely to occur with ulcerative colitis than with Crohn's disease, and may occur after trauma to the skin. It begins as pus-filled, raised, small bumps which become ulcerated. (This means that they lose the top layer of skin and become open sores.) Even though pus is present, there is no infection. Although the exact cause of pyoderma gangrenosum is still not understood, this condition must be brought to your physician's attention *immediately* since effective treatment of IBD often promotes healing of the ulcerations. Local medications may be helpful in preventing infection. Pyoderma gangrenosum is, at times, unresponsive to medical treatment. Fortunately, if surgery is performed to remove the diseased intestine, the skin disease usually disappears completely.

Perianal Problems

Perianal disease (inflammation occuring around the anal region) is more commonly associated with Crohn's disease than with ulcerative colitis. Local skin irritation may be the only problem, or one of several other local conditions may develop. These include internal and external hemorrhoids, fissures, and fistulas.

Hemorrhoids are swollen veins which may appear outside the anal sphincter (external hemorrhoids) or within the anal canal in a separate set of veins (internal hemorrhoids). A fissure is a small break in the lining of the anal canal which may extend into the lining of the rectum. Fistulas, which mainly occur in Crohn's disease, are connections that originate in one part of the intestinal tract and extend to a destination outside of the bowel wall. Fistulas surrounding the anal region usually have their origin in the tissues just inside the anal muscle or sphincter. The fistula burrows within the surrounding tissues and exits through the skin near the anus. The route that a fistula takes is known as its tract, and the tract may be single or branch into multiple tracts. In some cases, fistulas and the damage they cause in underlying tissue can be quite severe and require medical treatment. Fortunately, recent experience with the drug metronidazole has been very encouraging, and fistulas will often heal when the patient is treated with this medication. After the medication is stopped, however, the fistulas may recur. Other medications such as sulfasalazine, broad-spectrum antibiotics, and immunosuppressive agents may also be helpful.

Other than the treatment prescribed by your doctor, there is a great deal that *you* can do to reduce the discomfort and possibly even the development of some perianal problems. In general, people with IBD have frequent loose bowel movements that tend to be irritating to the anus and its surrounding tissues. Even if the specific conditions mentioned above are not present, local irritation may still be a nuisance. Here are a few guidelines for minimizing the skin problems surrounding the anal region.

First, the extent to which loose bowel movements can be changed to formed movements will make skin care and perianal care easier. Sometimes, bowel movements can be given more form by the use of bulk-forming substances such as finely powdered psyllium seed which is available under a number of trade names. This material is a hydrophilic meaning that it absorbs water. The water-absorbing property removes some of the liquid within the intestine and adds bulk to the stool. Most people tolerate powdered psyllium seed with no difficulty; some experience bloating or gas especially when the product is used for the first time. Frequently, the unpleasant sensation of bloating, distension, or gas diminishes with time. A bulkier stool may also reduce the symptoms caused by hemorrhoids, fissures and fistulas.

If diarrhea continues to be a problem, discussion with your physician may be needed. A number of effective anti-diarrheal agents are available to reduce the frequency of watery diarrhea, thus limiting perianal skin problems.

Some simple remedies may be useful to reduce local irritation. Cotton balls should be used rather than toilet tissue. Cotton balls are about as soft as anything available, and can be used with a small amount of soap and water for cleansing. The soap, as with tissues and cleansing solutions, should be unscented and contain no chemicals. Irritated skin should be pat-dried and not wiped. A simple technique often used for babies with diaper rash is drying the skin with a hair dryer. If you use this method, be sure not to set the hair dryer too hot. Placing your free hand near the perianal area can help you choose the proper temperature. To keep the skin dry, apply a small amount of unscented talcum powder to the area, and dust a small amount into your underpants as well. If the skin around the anal region is severely irritated from leakage or frequent diarrhea, application of a small amount of zinc oxide ointment can help protect the irritated skin. Zinc oxide is a readily available non-prescription medication.

Additional measures may help in either preventing irritation or soothing slightly inflammed perianal skin. Sitting in a warm tub once a day is helpful. In general, the softer the toilet tissue used, the better. It is wise to avoid tissue with any color, fragrance, or medication. Chemicals used in producing the color or the fragrance can themselves be irritating to the skin, particularly if there is already some inflammation. Cleaning solutions containing alcohol or chemicals should also be avoided. Commercially prepared wet wipes may contain a variety of chemicals including anesthetic agents. These chemicals can be "sensitizing," meaning that continued exposure to them may trigger a local reaction. Nevertheless, some people find wet wipes less irritating than dry tissue. Read the label and choose the ones with the fewest added chemicals.

There are a large number of over-the-counter medications advertised that might sound attractive to the IBD patient with perianal problems. Topical antihistimines, topical anesthetics, anti-itch preparations, cortisone with anesthetics generally should be avoided because they may produce local reaction with continued use.

If there are actual breaks in your skin (known as erosions), these need to be covered. Non-stick materials, such as Telfa, are superior to cotton or gauze because the cotton or gauze may stick to the exposed tissues. When the covering is removed, only non-stick materials will separate easily.

5 Caring For An Ostomy

Introduction

The decision to undergo ostomy surgery is one which is made by you, your gastroenterologist, your surgeon and others. The need for surgery depends on many factors. Many people feel that surgery is a very bad sign and that to have an ostomy means that somehow you have failed. This is not true. Surgery is related to the severity of your disease, the failure of medical treatment, the presence of complications such as fistulas, and the extent to which IBD interrupts your life and your ability to work and play. The type of surgery will also vary. Not everyone requiring surgery will need an ileostomy or any type of external stoma which requires the use of a pouch. For people with ulcerative colitis who require surgery, new surgical techniques have been developed which preserve continence (continent ileostomy, ileoanal anastomosis or "pull-through" operation). In Crohn's disease, surgery may require only the removal of the diseased segment of bowel and not the entire large bowel, so that an ileostomy is not necessary.

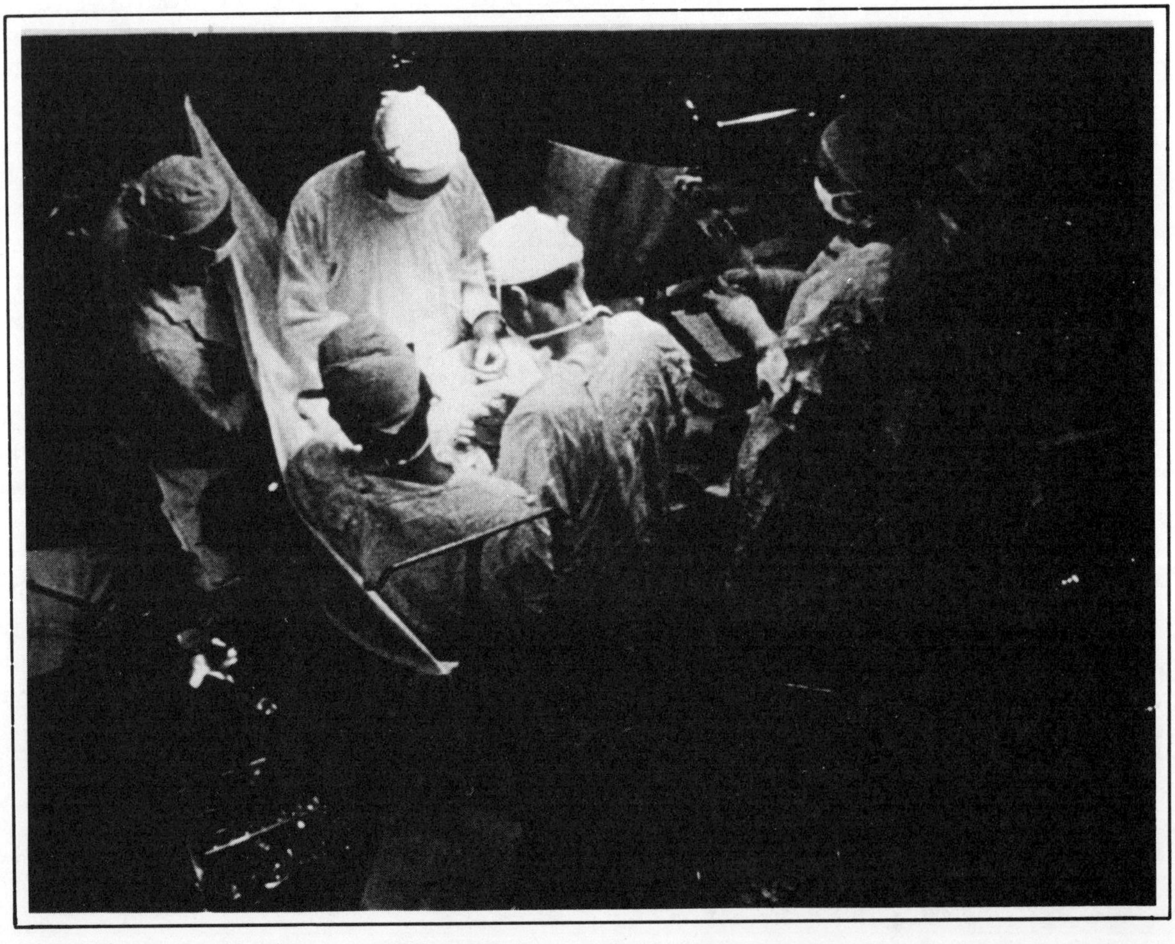

The purpose of this chapter is to discuss the impact of living with a conventional ostomy. The physical care and management of an ostomy is important. You will have to learn a new method of having bowel movements which is not "normal" and yet allows you to be in control of your elimination. The emotional and social concerns of people undergoing ostomy surgery are the key to learning to live with an ostomy. Even though you may have learned to live with chronic IBD, and even though you have reached an understanding that surgery is necessary for you, actually *having* ostomy surgery may be a very emotional time for you. The fear of the unknown and the lack of control all of us experience in hospitals only adds to all the reactions you may have when faced with surgery. This chapter will discuss some of the feelings which commonly occur before and after an ostomy. It is an honest appraisal of peoples' reactions when told they need the surgery and their successful adaptation to that surgery.

You will have to learn a new method of having bowel movements which is not "normal" and yet allows you to be in control of your elimination.

Many stories abound about ostomy surgery and living with an ostomy. The myths and misconceptions about ostomies would fill volumes. In the past, undergoing ostomy surgery was not considered a positive option. This was due to the lack of equipment, the lack of knowledge of health care professionals in caring for people after surgery, and the inability of most people to discuss bowel movements. Tragic tales of people being isolated from family and friends following ostomies are still heard. Fears of odor and leaking pouches are generally the basis for most stories you hear. In addition, people often respond to the notion of an ostomy in a manner which reflects their own emotions. No one would freely elect to have any surgery. Yet when faced with such a decision, the courage which people have to respond positively, to undergo necessary treatments, and to adapt successfully to the end results of surgery is amazing.

Feelings About Ostomy Surgery

When you have IBD, you usually know that ostomy surgery is a possibility. Perhaps your gastroenterologist mentioned it during your early years of treatment or during your remission when you discussed your options for living with these chronic illnesses. The thought of having an ostomy was probably hard. When actually faced with undergoing ostomy surgery, you may experience many feelings. Many reactions are normal and should be discussed openly with your physician, enterostomal therapist (E.T. nurse), and your family.

Adapting to and living with an ostomy means learning to manage the physical changes and recognizing the emotional reactions which you may have. It is normal to experience a time of grief for a loss which is real. There is the physical loss of a part of your body which cannot be seen, coupled with the physical change in your body and the addition of the stoma on the abdomen. There is no correct or right way to express your feelings about these changes. Some people go through stages of denying that anything is different; of anger that a cure or an alternative is unavailable; of depression which may be seen in changes in sleep and eating habits; and finally, of adapting and accepting the changes.

Accepting these changes does not imply that you like having an ostomy. It means that you can live with the ostomy. You need to be in control of the ostomy, not the other way around. You are still the same person you were before surgery. Accepting the change is, in part, realizing that you are the same and that you now have a different way of going to the bathroom.

Feelings About Your Body

A major concern is how your spouse or lover will accept you now that you are "different." The pouch which is present on your abdomen can be hidden by clothes, but during intimate contacts with your partner the pouch is evident and cannot always be hidden. The most important phase of intimacy is communication. Most people report that when they discuss the pouch, the stoma, and the changes in their body image, they find a loving, accepting partner. Partners may be afraid that they will hurt you if they give you a hug or put pressure on the stoma or pouch. You will need to teach them that normal pressure against the stoma is not painful or dangerous.

The most important phase of intimacy is communication. Most people report that when they discuss the pouch, the stoma, and the changes in their body image, they find a loving, accepting partner.

An ostomy should not limit your physical activities in any way. You can still be involved in sports as well as other recreational activities which you now enjoy. In fact, if you have had surgery and are now free of disease you may feel better than ever and be able to do more than before surgery. Or course, your age, the extent of disease, and any complications will effect the rate at which you recover from surgery and return to work and play.

The presence of the stoma and pouch *are* different. You will be very conscious of the pouch at first. You will notice every time stool collects in the pouch and you may find yourself emptying the pouch more often than necessary. This is a normal response to the newness of the pouch on your skin, the feel of the stool in the pouch, and fears of odor and leakage. As you become more active and more involved in other activities (as you recover from the surgery), you will become more accustomed to the pouch. You will learn when the pouch needs to be emptied based on its weight and feel, and you will be able to detect small signs which indicate it is time to change the system.

Talking About Your Ostomy

You will probably need someone to talk with about all the changes you are experiencing. Your E.T. nurse can provide many opportunities for you to ask questions and to share your feelings. You may also wish to meet someone who has had an ostomy and has successfully learned to live with the change. The United Ostomy Association (UOA) provides trained ostomy visitors who are available to come and talk with you before and after surgery. Either your E.T. nurse or your physician can make the arrangements to have the visitor meet with you. The UOA also organizes self-help groups in most areas where people meet to discuss facts about ostomies and to encourage open sharing of experiences related to living with an ostomy.

Some Ostomy Terms and What They Mean

Stoma—the visible portion of intestine that protrudes an opening on the skin. The stoma is formed by bringing the end of the small bowel through the abdominal wall and turning it back on itself, like a cuff. The stoma should be a bright red color and is moist to touch because the inner intestinal lining produces a mucus substance.

There are no sensory nerve endings in the stoma, so the sensation of pain is not present even though the red color makes one think it would be painful. The motor nerves in the stoma are still connected to the bowel, and the slight motion you will sometimes see in the stoma is the usual contractile or peristaltic motion of the bowel as it propels contents through the intestinal tract.

Ileostomy—an opening into the ileum or lower portion of the small intestine. The drainage from the stoma may be referred to as feces, stool, effluent, or bowel movements. The contents of ileostomy stool contain residual digestive enzymes which are normally present in the small bowel and which break down food products. The presence of these enzymes means that ileostomy stool is extremely irritating to the skin. The stool from an ileostomy occurs at unpredictable times. Most people report that they need to empty the pouch 4 to 6 times a day, generally after meals and before retiring at night. The stool will be very liquid right after surgery, but as your diet progresses to an unlimited pattern, you will notice that the stool will thicken. Unfortunately, you cannot predict when you will need to empty the pouch and for this reason you will need to wear an open-ended, drainable, odorproof pouch.

Pouches (Appliances, Bags)—the external collecting devices used following ostomy surgery. People have various reactions to each word since words have different meanings for different people. Pouches are odorproof, meaning that they will contain the normal odor of the stool until the bottom is opened for emptying. Pouches are also available in a variety of sizes, so that a pouch can be chosen for you which will fit your body contours and will not be visible under clothing (including bathing suits).

It is not necessary to wash or flush the pouch with warm water after each emptying. Some people like to flush the pouch once a day. The major thing to remember is to clean the spout with toilet tissue after each emptying. A clamp is used to close the bottom of the pouch and the edge of the pouch folds up into the clamp leaving an exposed edge. If stool is left on this edge or if your clamp is dirty, you may notice a minimal odor problem.

If gas is a problem, which it often is after surgery, several pouches are available which have charcoal filters. These filters deodorize the gas as it is released.

Ileoanal Anastomosis (with Reservoir)—a surgical option for people with ulcerative colitis when there is a minimal of perianal disease and excellent anal sphincter control. This surgery also involves the construction of a reservoir from the end portion of ileum. The ileum is then brought through a rectal cuff and sutured to the anus. The stool is eliminated in the normal fashion and continence is maintained by the sphincter muscles. The postoperative period does have some problems. Severe diarrhea has been reported for 6 to 12 months. Skin irritation around the anus is a problem because of the presence of the residual digestive enzymes. Some people have incontinence of small amounts of liquid stool at night. While this procedure is not for everyone, it does work well for selected people. It is important to have close follow-up care during the first year as the body adapts to the loss of the large colon and the creation of the small bowel reservoir. Good anal sphincter tone before surgery is a must.

Ileostomy

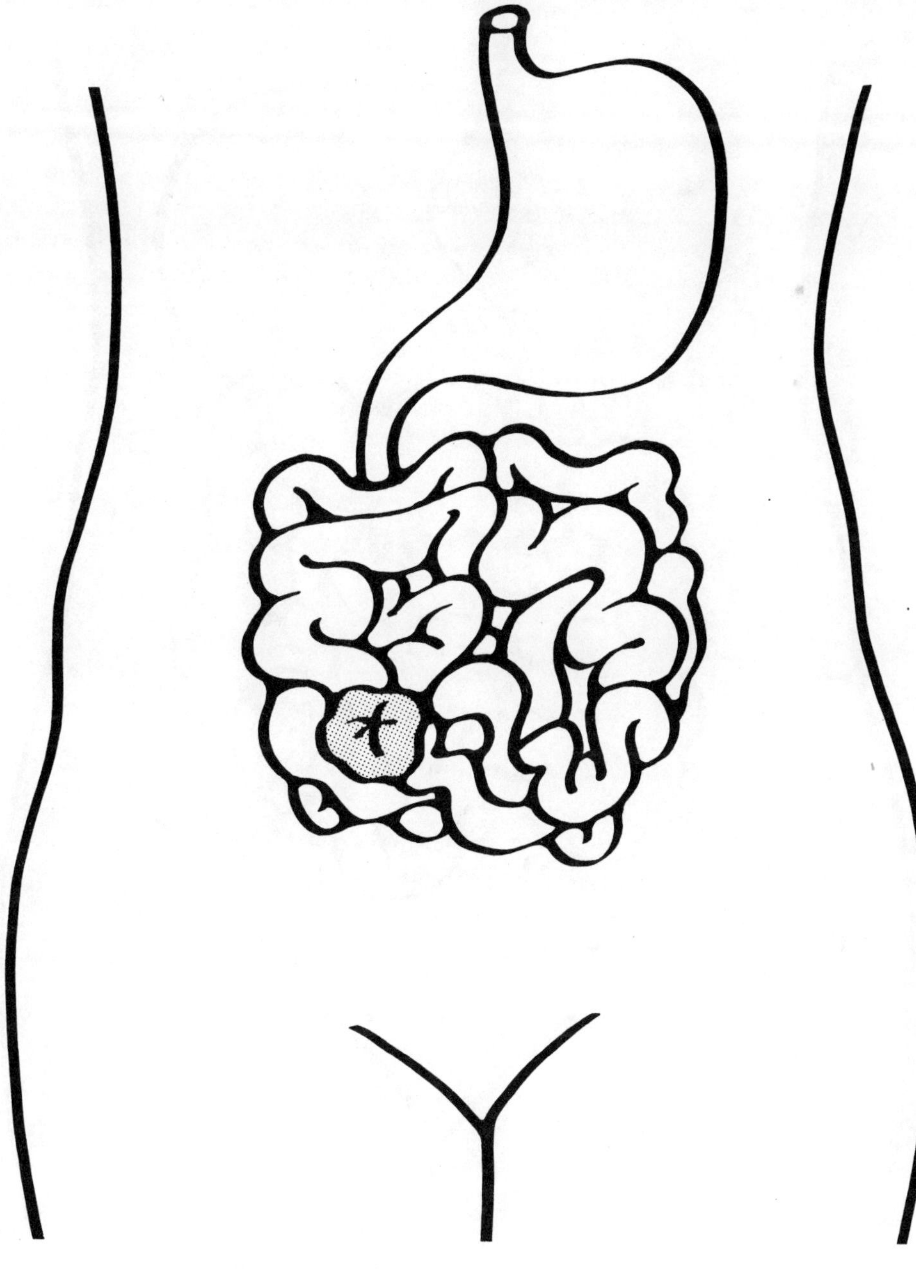

Reprinted with permission from the United Ostomy Association, Inc.

Continent Ileostomy (Kock Pouch)—a surgical procedure which is a possible option for people with ulcerative colitis. The surgeon constructs an internal pouch (reservoir) and valve from the end portion of the ileum. The opening through the abdominal wall is small and flush with the abdominal wall. Unlike the conventional ileostomy, there is no need for an external collecting device. A gauze covering or pad is worn over the opening to collect the mucus drainage. The continent ileostomy is emptied by the insertion of a catheter through the abdominal stoma into the pouch three to four times a day. Once a day, the person must use the catheter and a bulb syringe to flush the internal pouch with water.

Colostomy

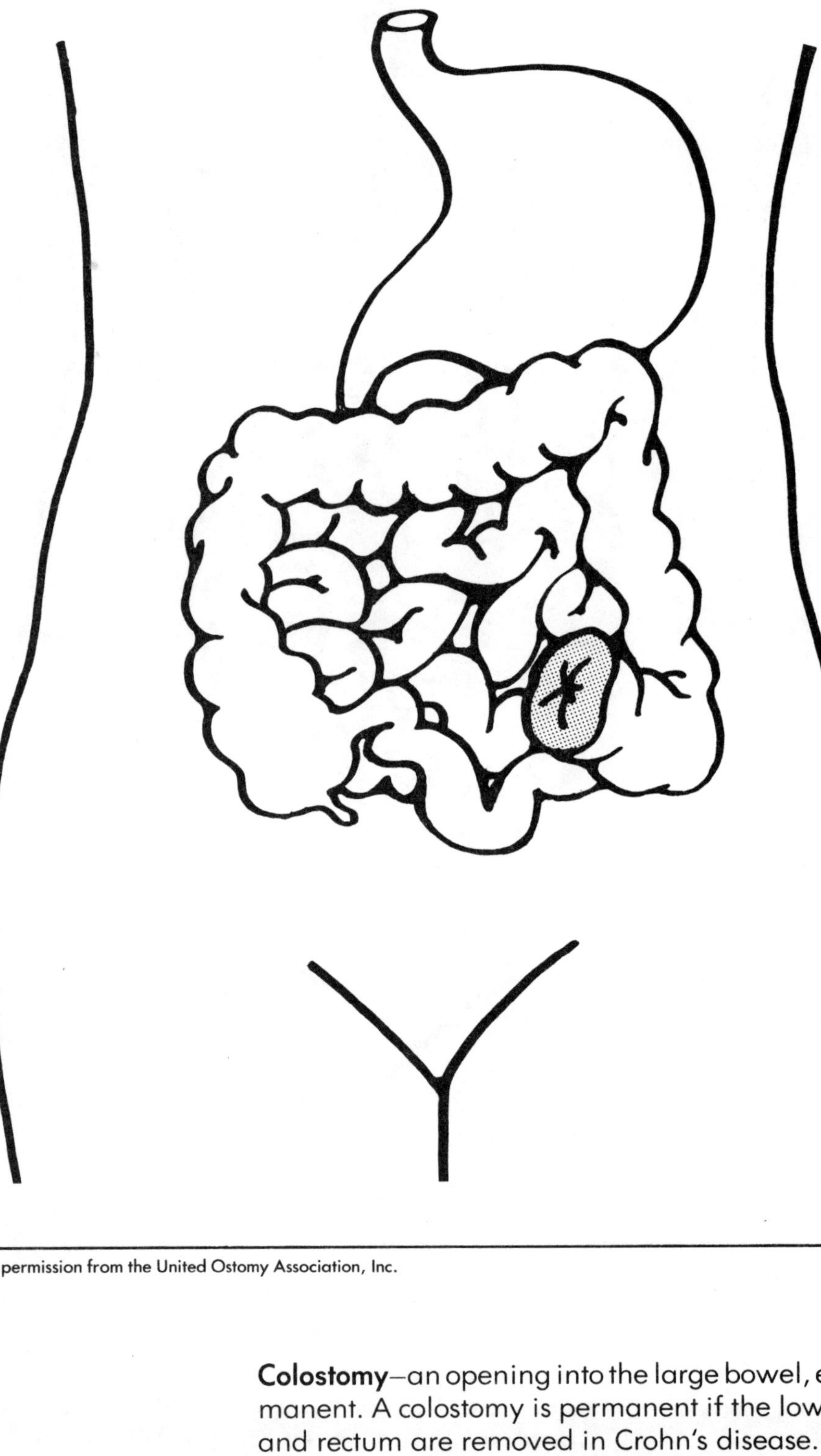

Reprinted with permission from the United Ostomy Association, Inc.

Colostomy—an opening into the large bowel, either temporary or permanent. A colostomy is permanent if the lower portion of the bowel and rectum are removed in Crohn's disease. The stool from a colostomy tends to be more formed than that from an ileostomy, and the residual digestive enzymes have usually been absorbed or deactivated by the time the stool passes through the ascending colon. You may hear of people with colostomies irrigating or giving an enema through the colostomy stoma to "control" their bowel movements. Generally colostomy irrigation is *not* recommended for people with Crohn's colitis. The disease process can recur and the bowel may be irritated by the irrigation process.

Ostomate—a general term used to refer to people who have undergone ostomy surgery. Many doctors and nurses will use it to refer collectively to people who have had ostomy surgery. As an individual, you can request that doctors and nurses not identify you as an ostomate. The aim of rehabilitation is to integrate the physical change (the ostomy) into your lifestyle, not to change your lifestyle to conform to having an ostomy. You are still a unique individual after surgery and the ostomy is only a small part of who you are.

Skin Barriers—products which provide a solid barrier to protect the skin. The most commonly used skin barrier is the pectin-based wafer. These wafers are useful in protecting the skin from breakdown and in promoting healing when minor irritations occur. The wafer should have an opening cut into it for the stoma. Many of the solid wafers are also available in paste form and can be used to fill in small creases or cover any exposed skin when the opening is a little too large. Some pouches are available with pectin-based wafers already attached.

Liquid skin barriers, referred to as skin sealants, are also available and are used to protect the skin under tape. Every effort should be made to keep your skin in excellent condition under and around the pouch.

Some Common Concerns About Ostomies

Odor is a major concern of most people who have an ostomy. Odor can be controlled and managed so that the only time you have a noticeable fecal odor is when you empty your pouch in the bathroom. Pouches are available which are odor-proof and odor resistant. Check the type of material your pouch is made of as you select any new equipment. Some people choose to take bismuth subgallate by mouth to control odor. With any orally ingested product, you should be careful about the amount and any possible side effects. Products are also available which can be inserted into pouches to minimize the odor. Charcoal filter systems are available to allow control of odor associated with the release of gas from the pouch.

Odor can also be a sign of a leaking pouch seal. If you have on an odor-proof system and you suddenly notice an odor, check your pouch seal and make sure everything is intact. Also double check your clamp and edge of the pouch for security of the seal formed by the clamp and for the presence of stool on the clamp or edge of the pouch.

Skin care is another area of concern. Peristomal skin refers to the skin around the stoma itself. The skin should be healthy and free of irritation. A good protective skin barrier and pouching system will keep your skin in good condition. It is important that you always protect your skin and that you change your pouch routinely before it leaks. Stool which sits on the skin underneath a pouch or skin barrier will cause a skin irritation.

Diet is an area that concerns every person with a new ostomy. For six to eight weeks following surgery, you may be kept on a low residue diet which eliminates bulky and hard to digest foods. You can then begin to add one new food each week until you have resumed a normal healthy diet. If some foods still bother you, just eliminate them from your meals. Some people recommend waiting a few weeks and trying a food again. They find that several months after surgery, certain foods are better tolerated.

It is important that you chew your food well, eat slowly, and avoid the use of straws. Chewing food well and eating slowly helps you digest your foods. It is particularly important with hard to digest, bulky foods such as corn, Chinese foods, and nuts. Drinking through a straw increases the air in your bowel which will cause more gas.

As we all know, some foods cause odor in the stool. Don't omit these foods if you like them. Just eat them in moderation. Rather than a pot of baked beans, try a small serving. Or eat all you want on an evening when you will be home and it won't matter if your ileostomy output is more active and you have more gas than usual.

Fluid intake is very important if you have an ileostomy. The large bowel is responsible for the absorption of water and salt from the stool. While the small bowel will absorb more fluid and salt when the large bowel is removed, you still need to make sure you take in enough fluids. During heavy exercise, when you perspire more, or if you have a "flu" with diarrhea and vomiting, you may lose more fluids and electrolytes than if you still had your large bowel in place. Gatorade and other high electrolyte drinks can be very helpful as supplements to keep you from having symptoms of dehydration.

Your Rights as a Patient

All people have rights, and people who happen to be patients have special rights. If you are having ostomy surgery, it is recommended that you see an enterostomal therapist, a nurse who has special training in working with people who have undergone ostomy surgery. The E.T. nurse is prepared to mark your stoma site before surgery to ensure a good location for maintaining a pouch seal; to choose appropriate pouches and skin barriers to contain your stool; to teach you and your family everything you need to know to be self-sufficient; and to help you work through the emotional issues which surround this surgery. You also have the right to have a properly constructed stoma in which the placement on your abdomen is considered before surgery and which is budded to make pouching more effective and secure. You also have the right to have an ostomy visitor. The main thing for you to remember is that you have the right to ask a lot of questions and to receive the answers you need to make decisions about your care.

In Case of Emergency...

It is recommended that you carry a Medic Alert card and/or bracelet with you. This is very important to let health care providers in emergency situations know exactly what type of surgery you have had and what it means in terms of your personal needs. While many people are familiar with colostomies, ileostomies are less common and the two are often confused. Continent ileostomies and ileoanal reservoirs are so new that Medic Alert Cards are even more important for this group of people. Medic Alert information may be obtained by writing the Medic Alert Foundation, P.O. Box 1009, Turlock, CA 95381-1009.

For Further Information...

The International Association for Enterostomal Therapy (IAET) publishes the *Directory of Out-Patient Ostomy Resources*, a listing of enterostomal therapy nurses who accept referrals of people with ostomies, for teaching, consultation, and rehabilitation. This reference book is available for a purchase price of $6.00.

Please contact:

International Association for Enterostomal Therapy
5000 Birch Street, Suite 400
Newport Beach, CA 92660
714-476-0268

Coping With an Ileostomy: Personal Perspectives

John C. Steers
Program Manager, Community Programs
IBM Corporation

My ulcerative colitis was diagnosed in June 1980. Four and a half years of accelerating illness followed. Despite the concerned attention of my family and two fine gastroenterologists, despite two hospitalizations, medications, treatments and tests of all kinds, the trend line on my chart was clearly going downhill.

Early in 1984, I was back in the hospital for the third time. More than ever before I was aware of the somewhat higher potential for colon cancer of those of us with ulcerative colitis. I knew to watch with my doctor for signals that would tell us that I had become part of the high risk or "pre-cancer" category. The sign we watched for was dysplasia, alteration in the cells of the colon, characteristic microscopic changes that occur in the cells lining the colon.

My third stay in the hospital included another colonoscopy. Multiple biopsy samplings were taken as part of this test to provide, among other things, the answer to the dysplasia question. This time the answer for me was unwelcome. The colonoscopy identified severe dysplasia and as a consequence major surgery had to be considered.

The decision to have surgery was an easy one for me to make. Suffice it to say that abdominal pain, chronic diarrhea—sometimes twenty times a day—bleeding and low grade fever, are what I dealt with as best I could. The worst of it was the embarrassment of having this "unmentionable bathroom disease," having to always know where the bathroom is, whether shopping, at the movies, or on customer calls. After a number of years of this kind of thing, I was willing to at least consider a trade-off action.

Some time before this third hospitalization, with my wife's support and advice from my gastroenterologist, I had already made a contingency decision: if and when signficant dysplasia appeared in my colon, I would have surgery—a total proctocolectomy with a standard ileostomy. In the hospital for less than ten days, at home for almost three weeks, I was back at my office shortly thereafter.

"You need the hand of someone who has experienced exactly what you are going through, who can tell you what it's like, who can be your model and personify the hope you have for your own recovery."

What did I learn from all this? What lessons learned would be of any interest to unhappy people who might find themselves in the same rocky boat I climbed into back in 1980?

There are a number of things:

- Choose a doctor you can have confidence in. Ask your doctor all the how's and why's you have on your mind. Don't hold back.
- Be sure you understand not only what your medications are but what their side effects are as well. Sometimes the cure seems worse than the disease.
- Before a major decision or major surgery, go for a second opinion. Your doctor should understand and even help you find the right person.
- Buy a book. It's NFIC's *Crohn's Disease and Ulcerative Colitis Fact Book*. It tells it like it is and in terms you can understand. As I went to the hospital for my operation I had it in my hand. It was, for me, a principal coping tool. It is complete, comprehensive and on target.
- Get some help. Those of us with these problems sometimes need more than even the most supportive of families can give. You need the hand of someone who has experienced exactly what you are going through, who can tell you what it's like, who can be your model and personify the hope you have for your own recovery.

  As I went into surgery, there were a number of reasons for my success in coping with ulcerative colitis. One was a man, a stranger, someone who had been in my shoes not too long ago and offers his time to help people like myself, needing ostomy surgery. My gastroenterologist asked if I was interested and gave this man my telephone number. The man called me and that evening was with me, in my home, for three hours. Here was an ostomate, a country club manager, a father of young kids, an athlete, who personified my hope for myself in the months ahead. If he could make it, I could too.

Last spring I joined a mutual help group sponsored by NFIC. About 15 of us met informally once a week for eight weeks. It was a rewarding program and enormously helpful. We pooled our experiences and feelings about all issues related to our illness without embarrassment. We helped each other, and in the process, helped ourselves.

- After surgery, and even before, seek out an enterostomal therapist. Ask your doctor, since there well may be one affiliated with your hospital or at least near by. Such people are an invaluable resource as you learn to care for your new body, your stoma, your alternative means of handling body waste. When you need help with post-operative problems or just information about appliances and new developments in the field, your best bet is your enterostomal therapist.

In all of this I am the lucky one: I am cured. Of course nothing is as easy as that, and a bag at my side will remind me of this for the rest of my life.

Finally, there is a challenge for all of us who have IBD, regardless of its form or status. It's the battle for control. Are you in charge, or is the disease? Do you indulge in self-pity and preoccupation? I do sometimes. So my strategy is simple. I try to stop looking back so much and get on with the rest of my life.

Donald P. Binder

Acting Director of the United Ostomy Association, Inc.

"Living with an ileostomy is no big deal." These words are easily spoken by someone who has had this surgery for 26 years. As time passes and one gains experience, an ileostomy becomes merely a part of one's daily routine: bathing, grooming, eating, toileting. Emptying an ileostomy appliance is just a different manner of accomplishing one's bathroom needs. Changing the appliance is planned, just as periodic shampoos are planned.

This seems like a nice neat package, but it does not arrive on day one following the surgery. Life in general has its annoyances: bad days at work, stressful personal situations, colds or minor ailments during the year, traffic tie-ups. The ileostomy will cause some trying moments: it requires attention as you are hurrying to get somewhere; the appliance becomes dislodged while dining at a nice restaurant; a noise from the stoma attracts attention at a cocktail party or during an intimate moment. These disruptions seem more devastating and embarrassing because they do not happen to everyone. Everyone does not have an ileostomy and, in fact, most people do not understand it very well even if they recognize the term.

The physical part of living with an ileostomy should not be a problem today. Better surgical techniques, better care and teaching in the post-op stage, better equipment and supplies, availability of products, information from the supply sources, the experience and support of the United Ostomy Association (UOA) chapters, and published information all combine to make the physical care easy to accomplish. There are also numerous resources for coping with the psychological part of having an ileostomy, but psychological stability is basically an individual matter. Some will adjust easily from the first day, others will take longer.

''Accepting the ileostomy takes the same positive attitude and self-concept as accepting your height, coloring, and other physical attributes.''

Accepting the ileostomy takes the same positive attitude and self-concept as accepting your height, coloring, and other physical attributes. Physical characteristics cannot be changed; for most, having an ileostomy is also something that can't be changed. One young woman remarked at a recent UOA Conference that if she could change one physical part of herself, it wouldn't be her ileostomy!

The reason for having an ileostomy can be a big factor in acceptance. In a case of someone who has coped long and tediously with ulcerative colitis or Crohn's disease, the immediate relief from the illness can be the beginning of a whole new life.

When one is first told that an ileostomy is necessary, the news may be devastating. Each person's concerns may be somewhat different, depending on the situation. Young single people are concerned about finishing education, starting a career, marriage, activities. Married people worry about whether their spouses will accept them, whether they will be able to have children, how the children will feel, if they can continue their jobs. All are legitimate concerns, but ones that are usually resolved with experience and time.

The encouragement that "you'll be all right" from medical staff and other well-wishers is often rejected or politely filed away. "That's easy for you to say, you're not lying here wearing an appliance."

The road is rarely straight and smooth. There will be some rough spots, but one has to be careful that the ileostomy isn't used as a crutch. Many times a stoma has been blamed for things that happen, just because it is there. The stoma is blamed for rejection, divorce, job loss, not getting a job. To be sure, these instances occur, but not as often as blame is given.

One advantage an ileostomy has over other disabilities is that no one will know you have it unless you tell, or unless the appliance is seen. Whom to tell, when to tell, and how to tell are concerns that ostomates approach with much trepidation. One young panelist at a UOA Regional Conference stated; "I tell when discovery is imminent." Some ileostomates tell no one outside of their immediate family. Others tell even casual acquaintances. Ileostomates who are actively involved in an ostomy chapter will find it difficult not to tell eventually. But these people usually have no problem with it or they probably wouldn't be so involved.

It is normal to be nervous and apprehensive when facing this situation, especially when telling someone you really care about. Explain that you are nervous, so it isn't misinterpreted. If you are not positive about your self-image, others will probably not be positive about you either.

Then there are those intimate moments. Whether it is the first time with someone or the first time since the surgery, you want it to go well, to be special. You want to be assured that the ileostomy is okay. Ileostomates have devised ingenious cover-ups using appliance covers, split crotch panties, and cummerbunds. Some are not that concerned and do not cover the appliance. Even if it doesn't go as well as planned, all is not lost. How you and your partner treat the situation is important. Talk about your feelings and concerns, enjoy the closeness, and try again later. The important thing is that you accept each other.

Ileostomates can participate in sports, but a major concern is showering in an open area. The appliance is in plain view of others. Sometimes there is no easy alternative. I faced the situation when I thought about playing basketball in a community league. There were three choices: wait until everyone else had showered, not take a shower, or not play basketball. Since I wanted to play, none of the choices were good solutions. So I played and faced the music. I stood with my back to the others as much as possible, but I did get some questions from the guys who played on my team, and there were some quizzical looks from others. But I would have been curious if I were not the ileostomate and saw someone wearing an appliance.

One trait that ileostomates (along with other ostomates) show is a remarkable display of positive attitude. This has been noted time and time again by people attending chapter meetings or ostomy conferences. Ileostomates also express a change in their priorities since the surgery. Having faced a serious, sometimes life-threatening situation, and coming out of it so well helps them focus on the important things in life.

You would not choose to have an ileostomy if it weren't necessary. For some, there are other choices today. But if the surgery is necessary and an appliance must be worn for the rest of your life, it is merely an adjustment. An ileostomy can be accepted in the same way other life situations are accepted. Or it can be rejected and fought. It's a matter of self image, attitude and priorities. The response is within each of us.

II

Fighting Back

6

People With IBD And How They Cope

In this chapter, people with IBD tell their stories. There are some with ulcerative colitis, some with Crohn's disease, some who have had surgery, some who continue to be treated medically. There are adults and young children. What they have in common is their willingness to share the details about their struggles with IBD, and the philosophies they have developed as a result.

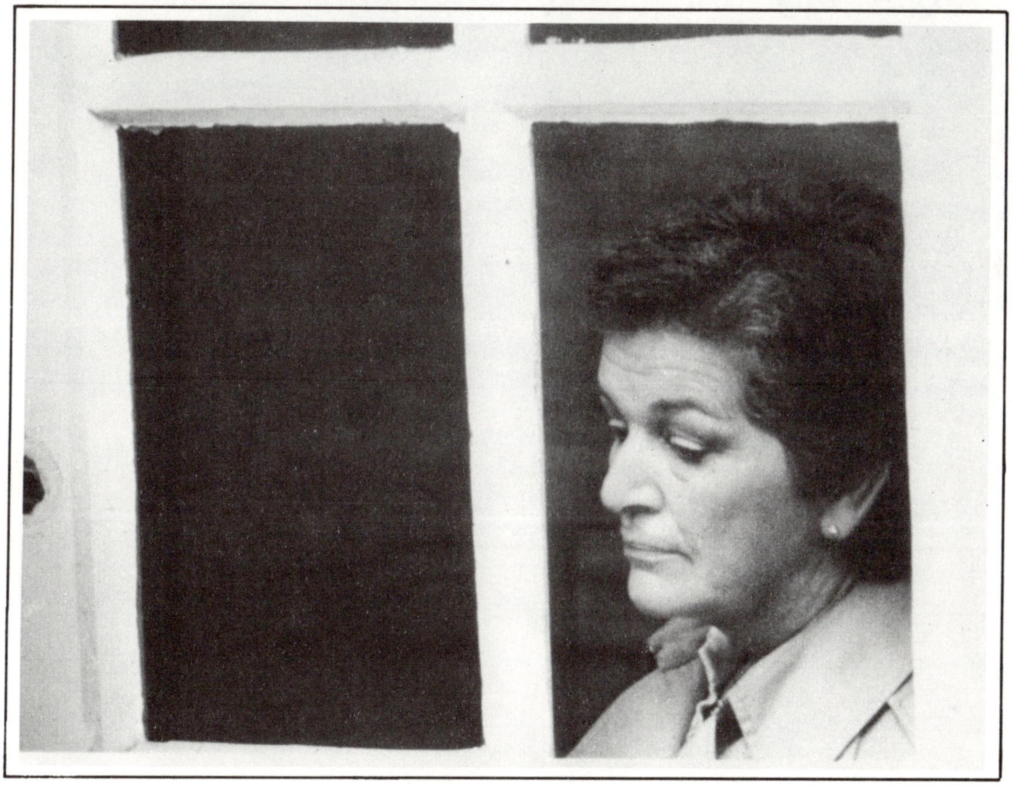

Not everyone with IBD will be as affected by the disease as some of them have been. Many will be fortunate enough to be able to treat Crohn's disease or ulcerative colitis as an inconvenience to an otherwise normal lifestyle. Often, however, those who are sicker are forced to come to terms with a disease which threatens to control every aspect of living.

In this chapter, you will meet both kinds of people with IBD, and several in between.

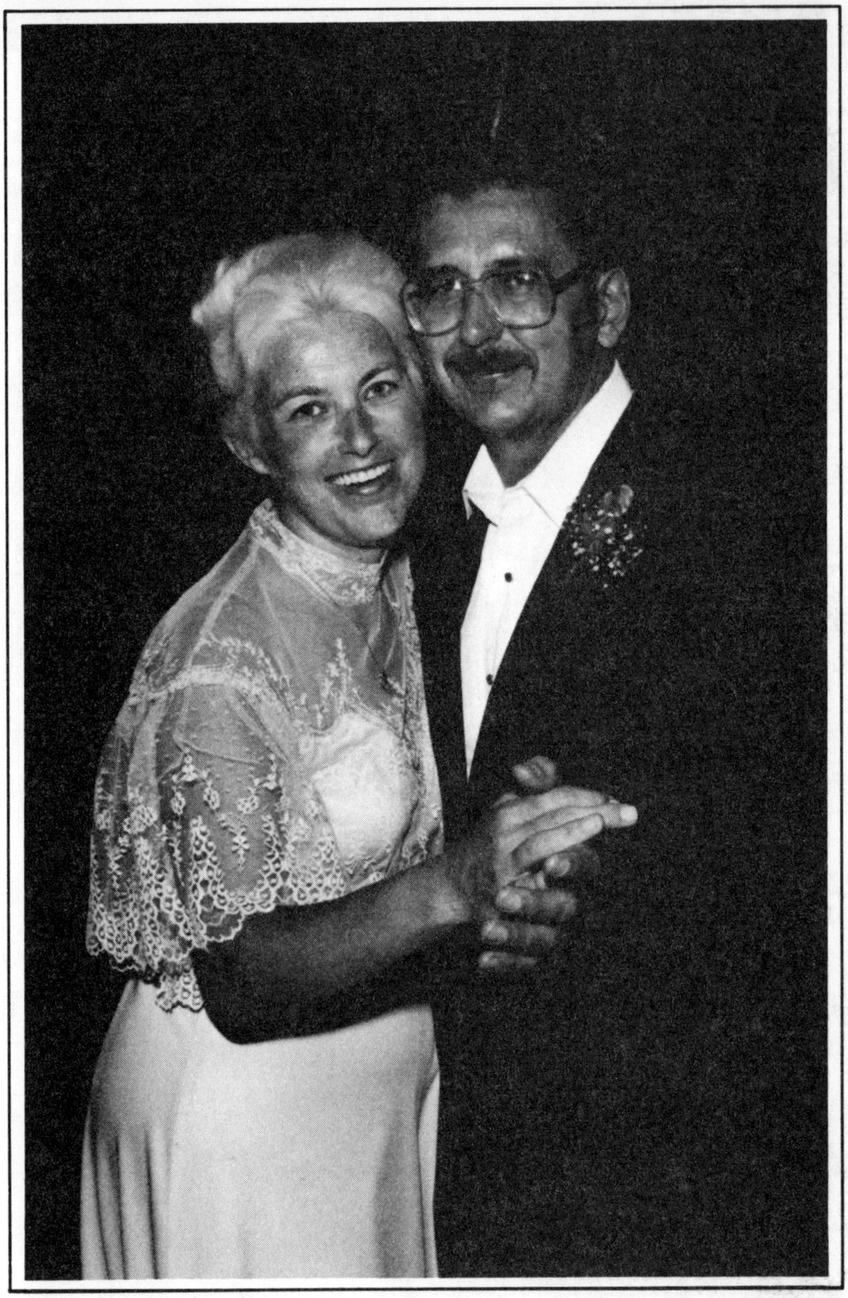

Beverly and Russell McCann

Russell McCann
Des Plaines, Illinois

"I'm a person, not a patient and can do just about anything I want to. I definitely don't want or expect sympathy and I'm no longer too bashful to tell people about my feelings."

Russ McCann is also an optimist. At 48, after many flare-ups and three operations for Crohn's disease, he has made the mental adjustments necessary to take control over his life. How does he do it?

"For starters, I have a tremendous faith in God which definitely strengthens me and makes me a very positive-thinking person. Also, I'm lucky to have my own personal support team to call on. My wife, Beverly, my children, my doctors, and the Carmelite Sisters of Des Plaines are always there to help me 'fight back' when I feel down or very depressed."

"Some of my friends and relatives either couldn't or wouldn't understand my problem. . . . I now believe that's their problem, not mine."

The owner of a small heating business, Russ McCann talks about some of the low points. "There were many years of feeling guilty about not being able to take my family on vacations or spend as much time with them as I wanted. There was the time I almost lost my heating business because of my illness.

"Worst of all was finding out that my 13 year-old daughter also had Crohn's disease. She couldn't go to school and wasn't growing properly. But she made a complete turn-around, graduated from high school, and is now married and working full-time.

"There was also the worrying about some of my friends and relatives who couldn't or wouldn't understand my problem. My doctor helped me to start fighting back, and I now believe it's *their* problem, not mine."

The NFIC is a big part of Russ McCann's life. "Two years ago, Beverly and I joined the Carol Fisher Chapter. We attended a board meeting and were greatly impressed by the dedicated, hard-working members and the work they were involved in. Now we are board members and have helped start our chapter's support group."

Of particular importance to the McCanns is the knowledge that most of the money raised through their chapter's efforts goes to fund research. "When the cause and cure of IBD are found, we along with many others will enjoy the satisfaction of knowing we did our part."

Donna Lewis
Avery, California

Donna Lewis describes her IBD as a series of brick walls which she has learned to climb over in order to live the rest of her life.

Diagnosed as having ulcerative colitis at age 14, Donna winces when she recalls the painful experiences of her high school years. "I remember during my first period history class, asking for permission to use the restroom, the teacher granting it for awhile, then insisting that I was probably taking my cigarette break. I never smoked! So there I'd sit in class, praying for the urge and pain to go away. Many times it didn't, and then the whispering would begin as the odor filled the room. The bell would ring and home I would go, embarrassed and ashamed. Never a date!! When I learned to drive, things were fine as long as the lights were all green, but a red light put me in a panic."

"If only I could have talked to someone who had a pregnancy after an ostomy. . . I have never known such joy as that which motherhood brings."

About those painful years, Donna says, "I lived those nightmarish days alone, in the dark. I felt guilty; I felt dirty. Ulcerative colitis was said to be brought on by stress. My mother would follow me into the bathroom with a can of deodorizer. I was embarrassed. I married because I figured it was my only chance...at least he would stop at the restrooms. But he often said no one else would have me."

Donna's first marriage ended in divorce. According to Donna, she just kept putting one foot in front of the other until she met her present husband. "This time it was for real. This man believed I could do anything I wished by putting my mind to it. He never blinked at my trouble, he understood, he offered compassion."

Donna enrolled in Auction School in Kansas City, Missouri. After graduating second in a class of 325, she returned home to California. "I was sicker than I had ever been in my life. I remember grocery shopping and having to sneak out the door leaving a full basket standing, as there was no public toilet. If only I would have known others, a support group or organization to help me cope.

"This time surgery was a must. For the first time in my life I thought I was a real loser. Buy my husband was right by my side. We had only been married for 6 months! I had no children and I felt like I had lost the battle. I had fears and questions. 'Do you wear a 50-gallon garbage bag?' 'Are maternity clothes the only clothes you ever wear again?' 'What about swimming?' 'What about sex...a family?' As I lay in my hospital bed thumbing through a women's magazine, I ran

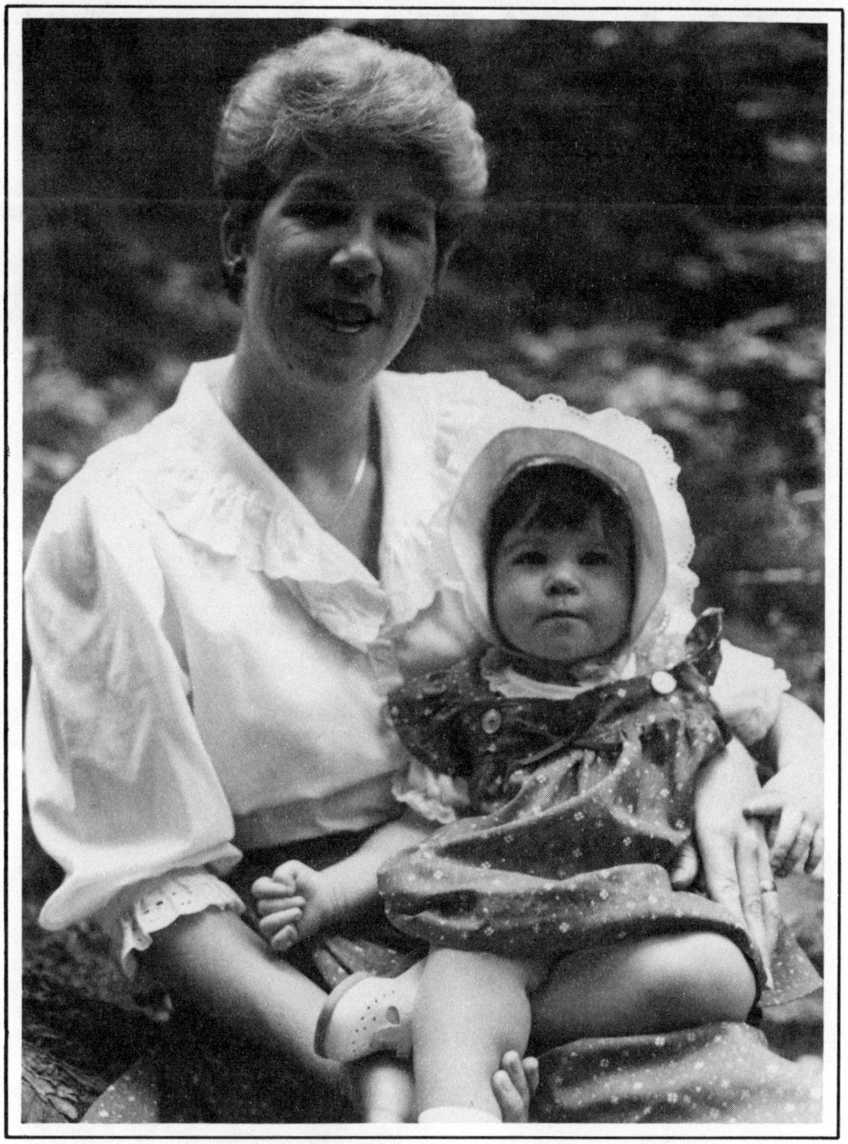

Donna Lewis and her daughter Ginny

across an ad for fashion undies. I thought I would never stop crying, but that was the end of my self pity. I had to get a hold of myself, face the facts head on, and go for it!"

After her ileostomy surgery, Donna bounced back quickly and performed her first auction just seven weeks after surgery. "Life began anew…I can't remember feeling better. Why didn't someone tell me or show me by example that life after ostomy surgery was normal. I swim, water ski, hike, horseback ride, jog, everything!"

Donna eventually became pregnant. "If only I could have talked to someone who had a pregnancy after an ostomy. I knew it happened, I was told by my E.T., but she had only read about it. I delivered a healthy 9 pound 5 ounce baby girl with no difficulty, and have never known such joy as that which motherhood brings."

Not once has Donna Lewis let her illness discourage her from moving ahead. She feels that with a positive attitude and with the support of loved ones, you can accomplish anything, you can climb over the walls.

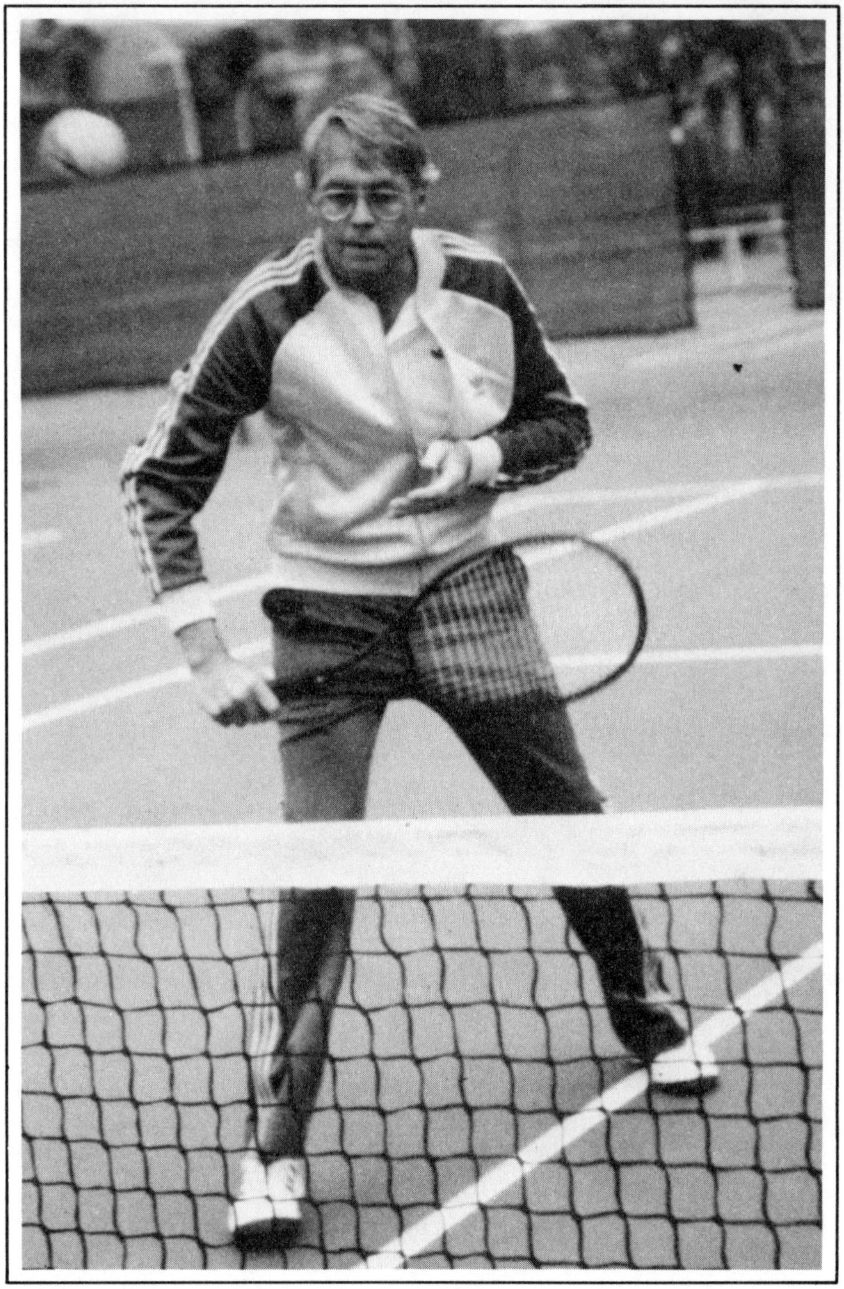

Vandy Christie

"I was traveling with my team but having real problems with stamina. My gastroenterologist told me to go directly to the hospital. When I got to the match, I told the team that they would be traveling to Minneapolis without me."

C. Vandy Christie
Evanston, Illinois

Vandy Christie's life has always centered around athletics. A life-long tournament tennis player, he was appointed men's tennis coach at his alma mater, Northwestern University, in 1975. He practiced with the team six days a week, traveled often to tournaments, and wasn't about to let IBD slow him down.

In 1981, Vandy suffered a relapse of his Crohn's disease, and in June of that year underwent the first of several operations which would leave him with only eighteen inches of small intestine. Weighing 128 pounds and having trouble even climbing a flight of stairs, Vandy returned to his coaching job at Northwestern. At the same time, he was faced with learning to eat again, and was subsisting on Ensure and elemental diets he would fix himself in a blender. But it wasn't enough.

"I was traveling with my team but having real problems with stamina. I knew the players sensed my struggle. On April 22, I saw my gastroenterologist who was aware of the problems I was having. He told me to go directly to the hospital, but I told him I had to coach a match in an hour, and had to leave in the morning for matches in Minneapolis. I agreed I was in no shape to travel. When I got to the match, I told my team I was going into the hospital and that they would be traveling to Minneapolis without me."

The evening, surgeons inserted a central catheter in a vein in Vandy's chest, and through the technique of total parenteral nutrition (TPN) he was able to "eat" again. Says Vandy, "I felt great after only 24 hours. My physician told me how I could have full-time home hyperalimentation without coming to the hospital! Thus I was introduced to TPN and it saved my life."

Each night at home, Vandy Christie connects the tubing from an IV bottle to the catheter implanted in his chest. While he sleeps, his body receives all the essential nutrients, vitamins and minerals he needs for life. Instead of being confined to the hospital, Vandy and his wife, Audrey, manage his entire nutrition program from home, with the help of one of the major firms now providing home health care services and equipment. Fortunately, the $200-per-day cost of Vandy's treatment is paid for by health insurance.

Thanks to TPN, Vandy's weight has returned to a normal 170 pounds. He eats when he feels like it, and has started playing tennis again.

"I play three or four times a week and I am able to work a full day, generally 10 to 12 hours. In January 1984, I stopped coaching and became the Director of Development for Athletics at Northwestern. My new job involves creating campaigns to raise money for athletic scholarships. I travel even more than I did while coaching, but I feel perfectly normal about it because I can take my TPN with me."

Vandy often visits people with IBD in the hospital. "I feel my experiences can help them overcome the effects of IBD. I am truly lucky to have met some wonderful people who have battled back from problems with IBD."

Vandy Christie is one of those people.

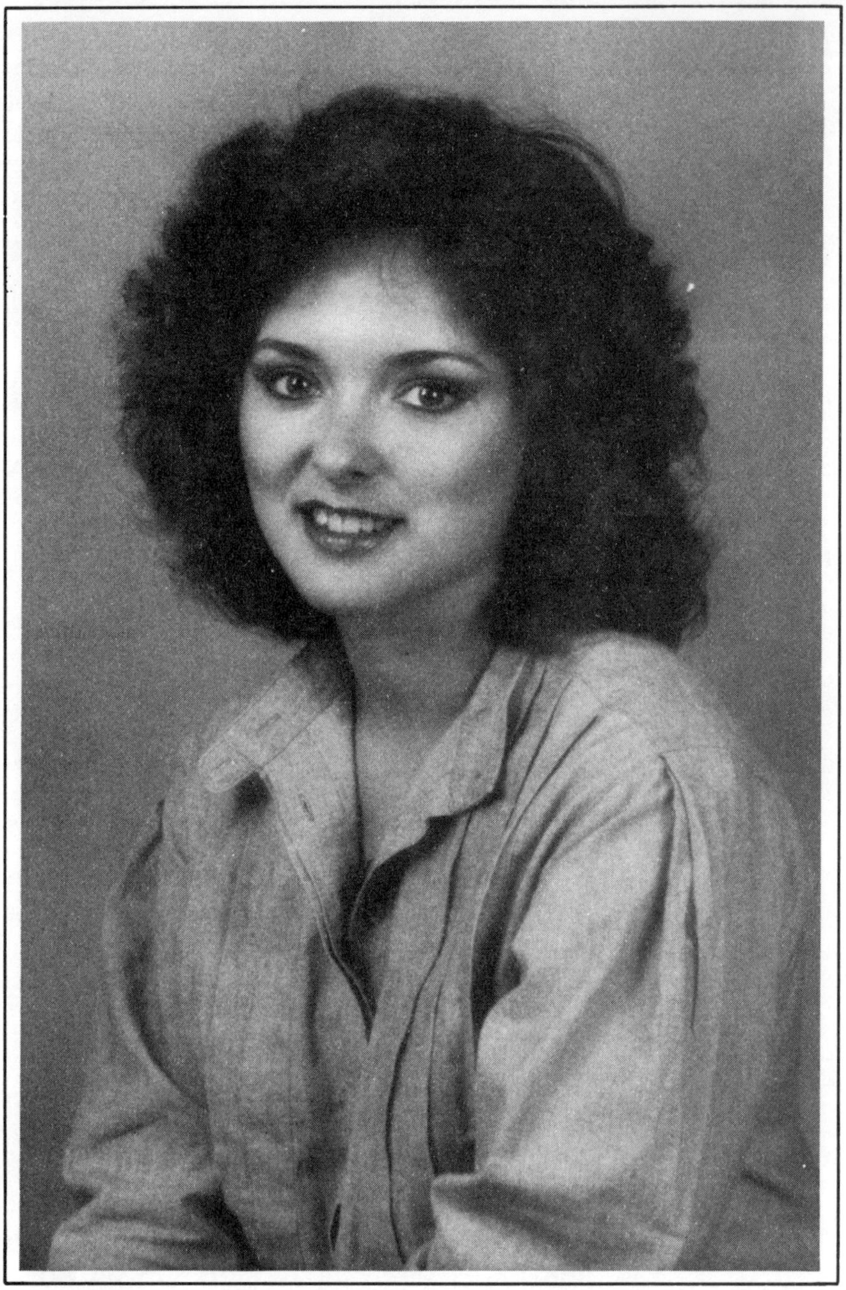

Caryn Murray

"My boyfriend always felt that if I tried harder, thought positively, and prayed, I wouldn't have colitis."

Caryn Murray
Woodridge, Illinois

Caryn Murray is doing well now. She has a good job as a waitress in an exclusive restaurant near Chicago. She has her family, her friends, and she has her health. But it hasn't always been this way.

At 26, Caryn says the hardest thing is "not being able to remember what it's like *not* to have ulcerative colitis." Even after 19 years, though, Caryn has kept the sense of humor that helped see her through the difficult high school and college years when, she says, "I felt like I was the only person in the world who had colitis."

Caryn's sense of humor is evident when she deals with her not-so-funny anxieties about making it to the bathroom on time. "At home and at work, if people cannot find me, I'm in the bathroom. It's a private joke at home, but at work it's another story. When I'm taking an order in the restaurant and I have a 'mad urge,' I make any excuse to leave the table. At times, I don't even have enough time to undress ...that's no way to live."

Caryn talks about her first accident: "I was 20 years old, in a fraternity house at college, with one female bathroom in a house full of 95 guys. My boyfriend's comment was, 'Don't you think you could have controlled yourself?' He always felt that if I tried harder, thought positively, and prayed, I wouldn't have colitis."

Caryn talks about turning down social invitations in college "because there would be a long car ride, and, psychologically, a bathroom wasn't within my reach...Another time I had an accident in the car on the way to an Earth, Wind, and Fire concert on Thanksgiving (nothing open), with my sister present. I always kid her that I would have committed suicide had I been on a date with a guy. I was so embarrassed."

Before taking her job as a waitress, Caryn was in restaurant management, working 12-14 hour days, five to six days a week. She became exhausted and at the same time her ulcerative colitis flared up again. Her doctors believed she might need surgery. She says, "Here I was, 25 years old and scared out of my mind. If only I could have talked to someone who understands, who knows what I'm going through, it would have helped a lot."

Recently, Caryn became active in NFIC's Carol Fisher Chapter in Chicago. "I want to help someone—anyone—especially someone in the hospital who's scared or doesn't understand. I want to be able to talk to them and let them know that someone else has the very same problem.

"Sometimes you get so aggravated and feel sorry for yourself. Why me? What did I do to deserve this? Now I realize how much better off I am than so many other people. You learn to live with your disease. That's the bottom line. It's a way of life."

Michael Medwar
Sharon, Massachusetts

Fourteen year old Michael Medwar's bedroom looks like a typical "boy's room," the kind you would see in a movie or home decorating magazine. Plaid bedspread, college banners, trophies. One wall has autographed photos of sports personalities, another all the sports schedules for the season. A huge pinup of Christie Brinkley in a very brief bathing suit covers a closet door. An Atari home computer and a small TV sit on his desk.

However, when you look again, there is something strikingly unusual. In one corner of the room there is a small pump and an IV pole with a plastic bag containing a solution. The "typical teenager" who uses this bedroom is not typical at all. Michael is on home TPN. Every night while he is sleeping the pump infuses the solution into his body.

Michael says, "I don't think about the future," and handles things as they come.

Michael has had Crohn's disease since he has been nine. He is using home TPN in the hope that it will provide additional calories to help him grow while giving his gastrointestinal tract a chance to rest and heal.

Michael and his parents learned the sophisticated procedures while he was hospitalized. When he came home he took responsibility for the setup every day. He says: "Now I'm a pro, but the first day my hands shook. First I was nervous, then it was something new, then it became a pain in the neck."

A nuisance, that's how Michael sees it now. Last year, before TPN, Michael missed lots of school. This year his attendance has been excellent.

Michael's disease and his present treatment do not keep him from doing the normal things a boy his age enjoys. After school, he does his homework, plays in the street with other kids, watches a little TV. He loves sports and says: "Right now, Carl Yastremski is my favorite athlete." He has a personally autographed photo of Carl Yastremski and a baseball autographed by every member of the Red Sox. He goes to church on Sunday, but not every Sunday. He looks straight at you through large dark eyes and makes it clear that he's not a "goody-goody."

Michael takes things in stride that would disturb most adults. He has a special sense of humor, almost a nonchallance. Yet one suspects it is an acceptance of how things are and a desire to do the best with them.

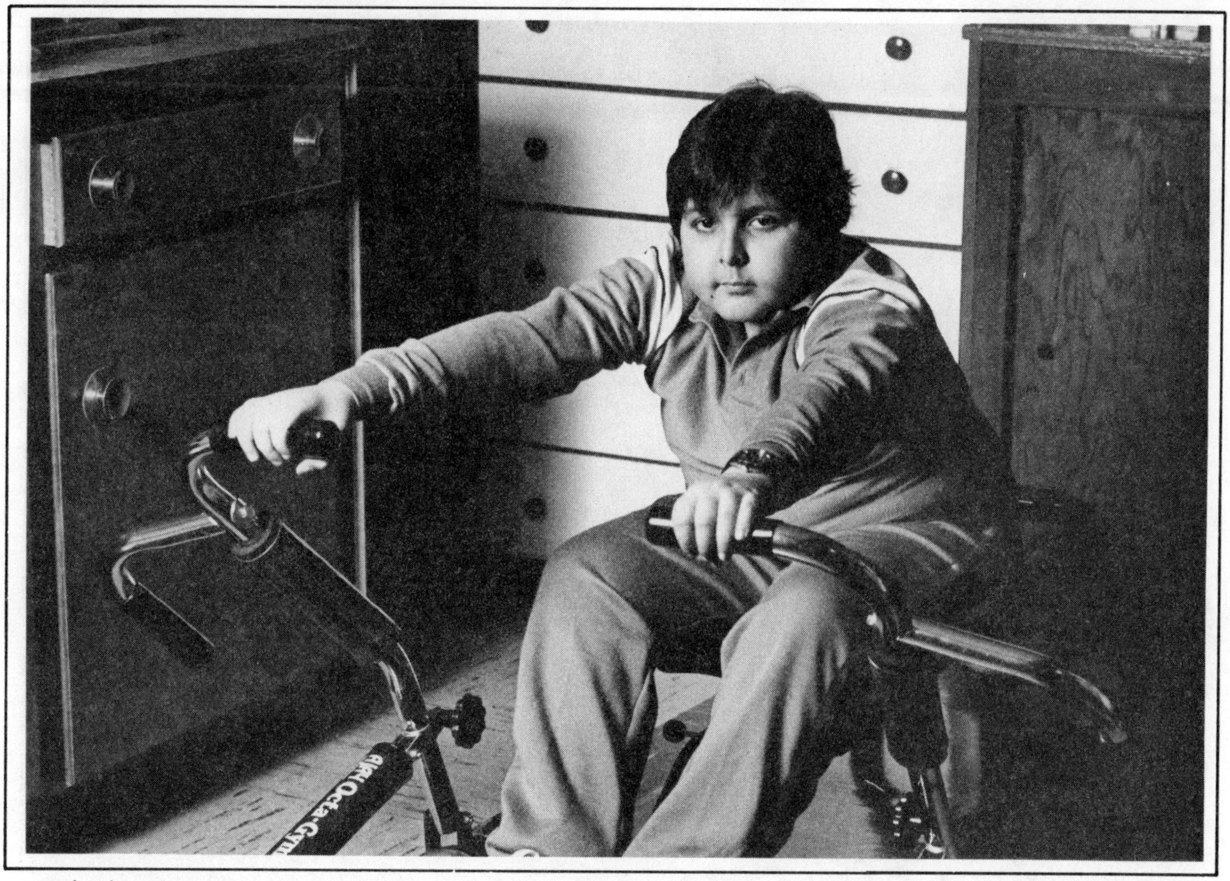

Michael Medwar—Photo by Irwin Sterbakov

He doesn't complain about the frequent doctor's appointments from Sharon to Boston, not eating even at holiday time, or the other restrictions. "My dad and I go to baseball games in the summer, but the cold is bad for me so we can't go to football games. It's O.K., we watch them on TV."

He doesn't complain, but Michael is unusually mature and one suspects his wry humor hides a very adult awareness. When asked about his plans for the future, he says: "I don't think about the future." Michael handles things as they come to him, in a most extraordinary way. His grace, humor, and concern for those around him are remarkable. A very special young man.

Reprinted with permission from The Newsletter, Greater Boston Chapter, NFIC.

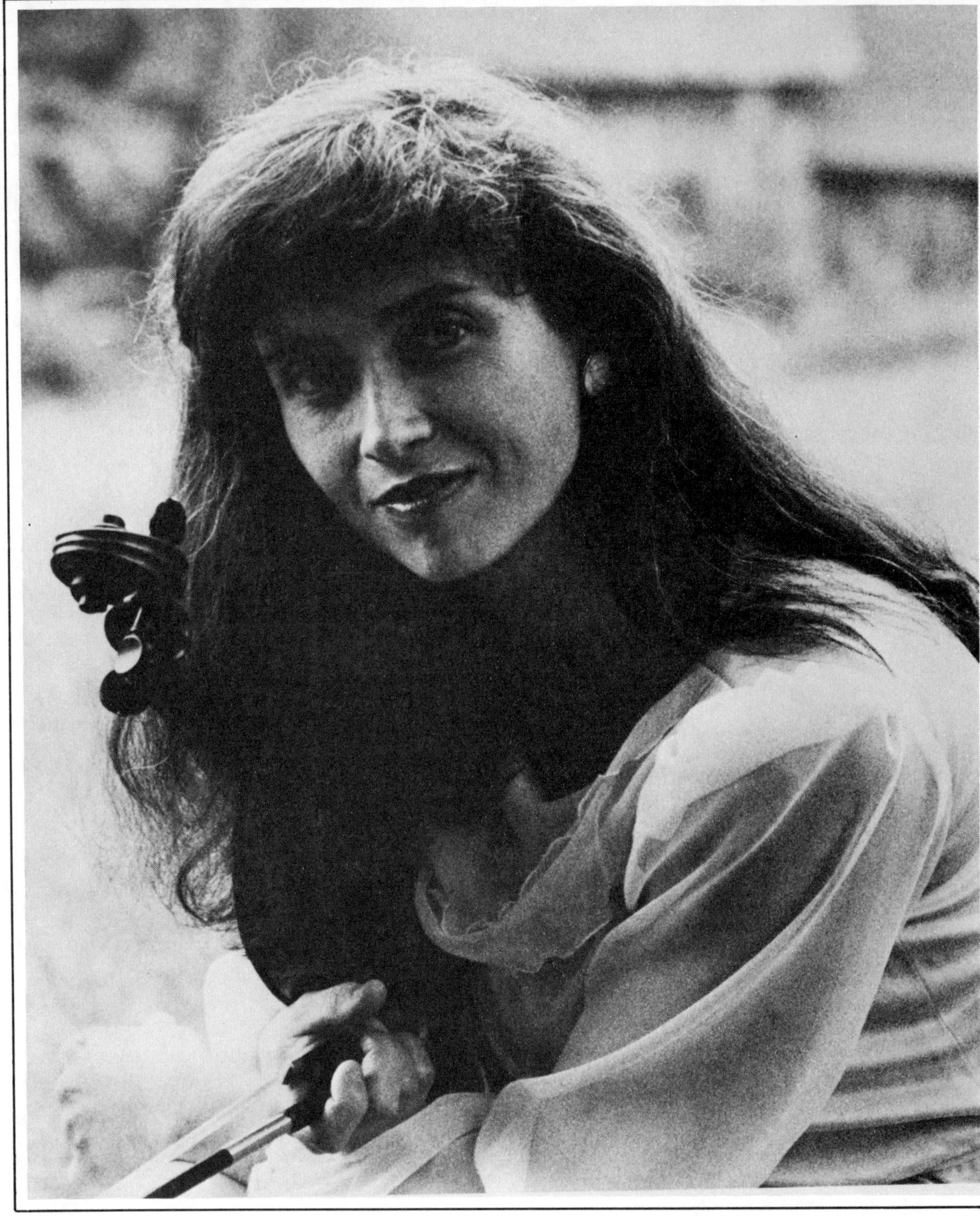

Rosemary Glyde

Rosemary Glyde
Golden's Bridge, New York

The Boston Globe called her "an exceptionally able and intense violist." But Rosemary Glyde is exceptional not only for her musical virtuosity, but for her courage and determination in overcoming the challenges of living with Crohn's disease.

Rosemary first became ill when she was 13. During the ensuing years, she suffered painful attacks and underwent surgery several times. However, Rosemary persevered in her studies, finally achieving her doctorate at the Juilliard School in 1975.

"When Rosemary first became ill," says her mother, "we never dreamed she would be able to achieve so much."

Advice from one of her doctors helped Rosemary overcome the emotional stress of living with Crohn's disease. When she was hospitalized, she would gaze out her window and comment on how much she wanted to be out in the world. Her doctor would simply point to her forehead and tell her that the world was in her mind. He would also tell her not to blame herself for the disease no matter how ill she felt. With these words in mind, Rosemary determined to push ahead, taking one day at a time, setting realistic goals.

Between 1976 and 1979, Rosemary was the violist for the Manhattan String Quartet. Since then, she has combined active careers as an ensemble performer, soloist and teacher. Recently she accepted an invitation to perform and lecture at the International Viola Congress at the New England Conservatory of Music in Boston.

Throughout her career, Rosemary has had to overcome setbacks due to Crohn's disease. She twice had to cancel performances with the Smetana Quartet because she had to be hospitalized. "Since I might not be well enough to perform in the next concert," she commented, "I give all my strength and energy to each performance."

Rosemary now lives in Golden's Bridge, New York, with her husband Noel Shumsky and her daughter Allison. Says her mother, Dorothy Glyde, "When Rosemary first became ill, we never dreamed that she would be able to achieve so much. I hope her story will inspire other young people with Crohn's disease or ulcerative colitis to try and realize their dreams."

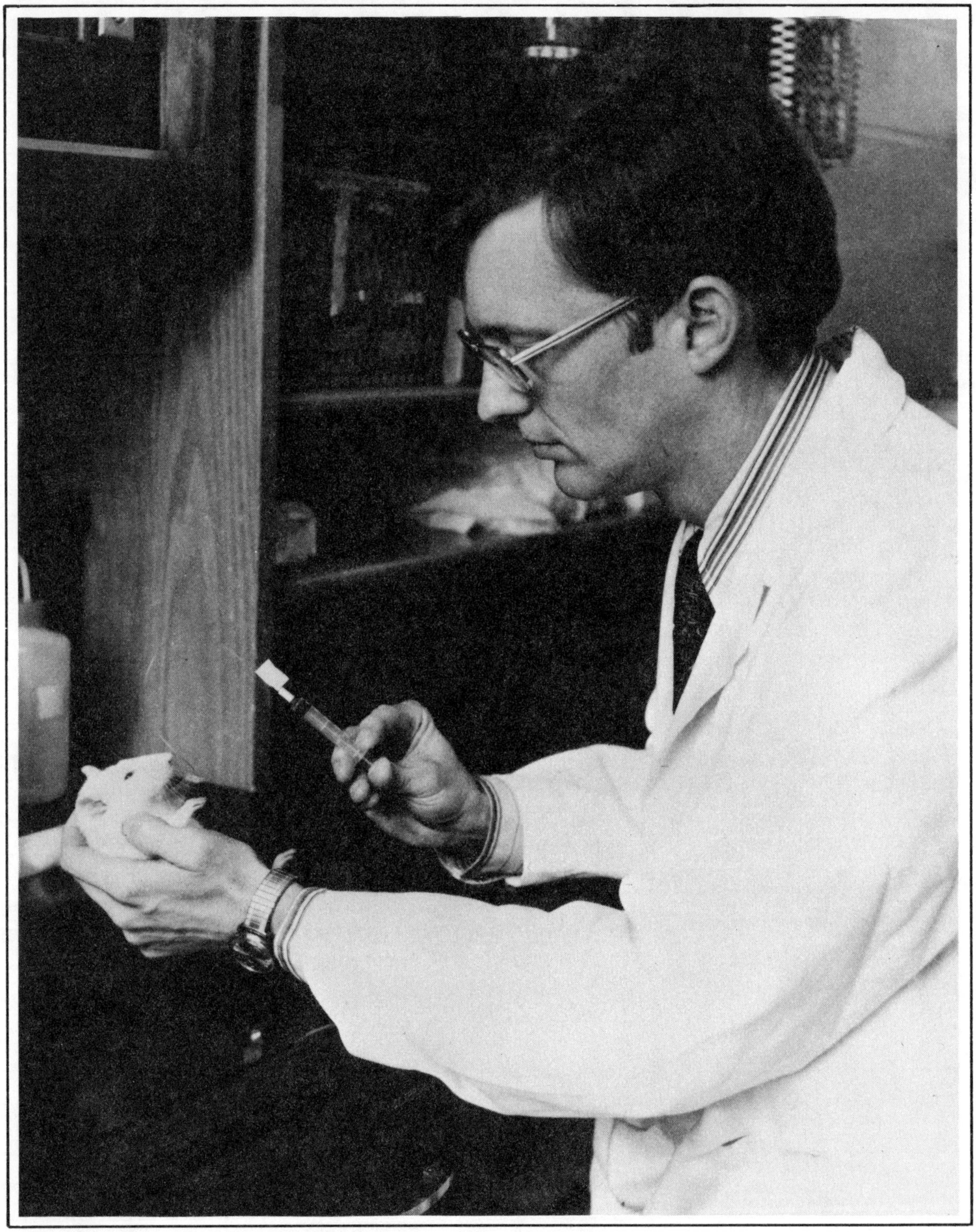

Balfour Sartor

R. Balfour Sartor, M.D.
Chapel Hill, North Carolina

NFIC's Research Training Awards Program was established in 1976 to encourage bright, young scientists to turn their careers toward the study of inflammatory bowel disease. Working under the sponsorship of established mentors in major medical centers, these young men and women bring fresh insight to the study of the nature and pathogenesis of Crohn's disease and ulcerative colitis. They are, quite literally, our best hope for the future.

"It's an asset for me as a physician to have been a patient with IBD. I know what it's like to be chronically sick."

R. Balfour Sartor, M.D., a 1981 recipient of NFIC's Senior Fellowship Award, is at once typical of these young scientists, yet different from all of them. Like many of the patients he treats at the University of North Carolina School of Medicine, Dr. Sartor has Crohn's disease. Stricken while a 21 year-old college senior and currently in remission, Sartor is candid about the effect of the disease on his career. "I think it's an asset for me as a physician to have been a patient with Crohn's disease. I *know* what it's like to be chronically sick," he says. Originally trained as a clinical gastroenterologist, Sartor feels his work with IBD patients together with his own experience with the disease have given him the motivation to pursue a career in research.

Balfour Sartor first contacted NFIC as a patient when he and his wife became involved in the Houston Chapter. After moving to North Carolina, Sartor became founding president of the Triangle Chapter, later its treasurer, and now serves as co-chairman of the Chapter Scientific Advisory Committee. He speaks softly in the accents of his native Louisiana, but beneath the exterior is a young man with a fierce determination. Once told that because of his disease he should give up the idea of going to medical school, Balfour Sartor now handles the varied roles of researcher, clinician, and chapter leader expertly. He is grateful for NFIC's willingness to give to him and to other unproved researchers the valuable experience they need to build a career.

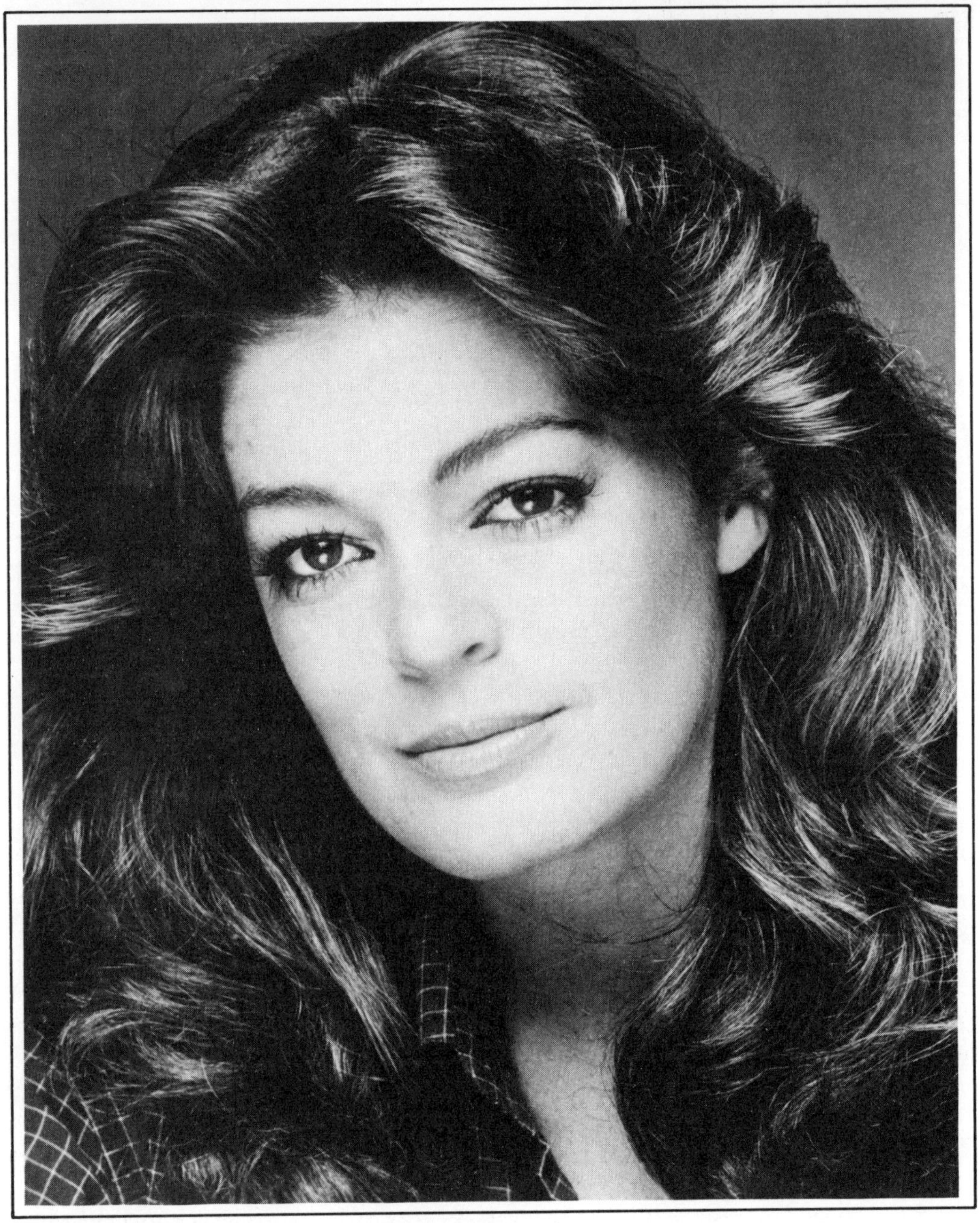

Donna Wright

Donna Wright
New York, New York

Donna Wright is everything you might expect a cheerleader for the New Jersey Generals football team to be: bright, attractive, outgoing, full of energy. When she isn't on the football field, Donna spends many hours each week rehearsing and taking dance and acting lessons.

Getting her job as a cheerleader was no easy task. She had to audition with 500 other young women, go through lengthy interviews and dance try-outs. Donna also had to battle a major flare-up of the Crohn's disease she has had since age 13. Finally diagnosed at the age of 19 after several resections, Donna was told by her physicians that she was "making herself sick."

Now at age 27, frustrated by myths and misunderstandings about a disease that was threatening to control her life, Donna has joined NFIC as a member of the National Sports Council.

Finally diagnosed at age 19, Donna was told by her physicians that she was "making herself sick."

As a spokesperson for NFIC, Donna has begun visiting New York area public schools. Wearing her red and white General's uniform with gold tassels around the waist and on the boots, she performs a few of her cheerleading routines while pop songs play in the background and the kids dance in their seats. Then she begins to speak about her battle with Crohn's disease and the auditorium suddenly becomes quiet. She tells the kids "how important it is to educate themselves about nutrition and health."

These days, Donna has her own health back, too. She has plans for an acting career and has a role in a newly-released film called "The New Girl," about an all-female college basketball team. Now that the myths about her disease are a thing of the past, Donna Wright can concentrate on her own bright future.

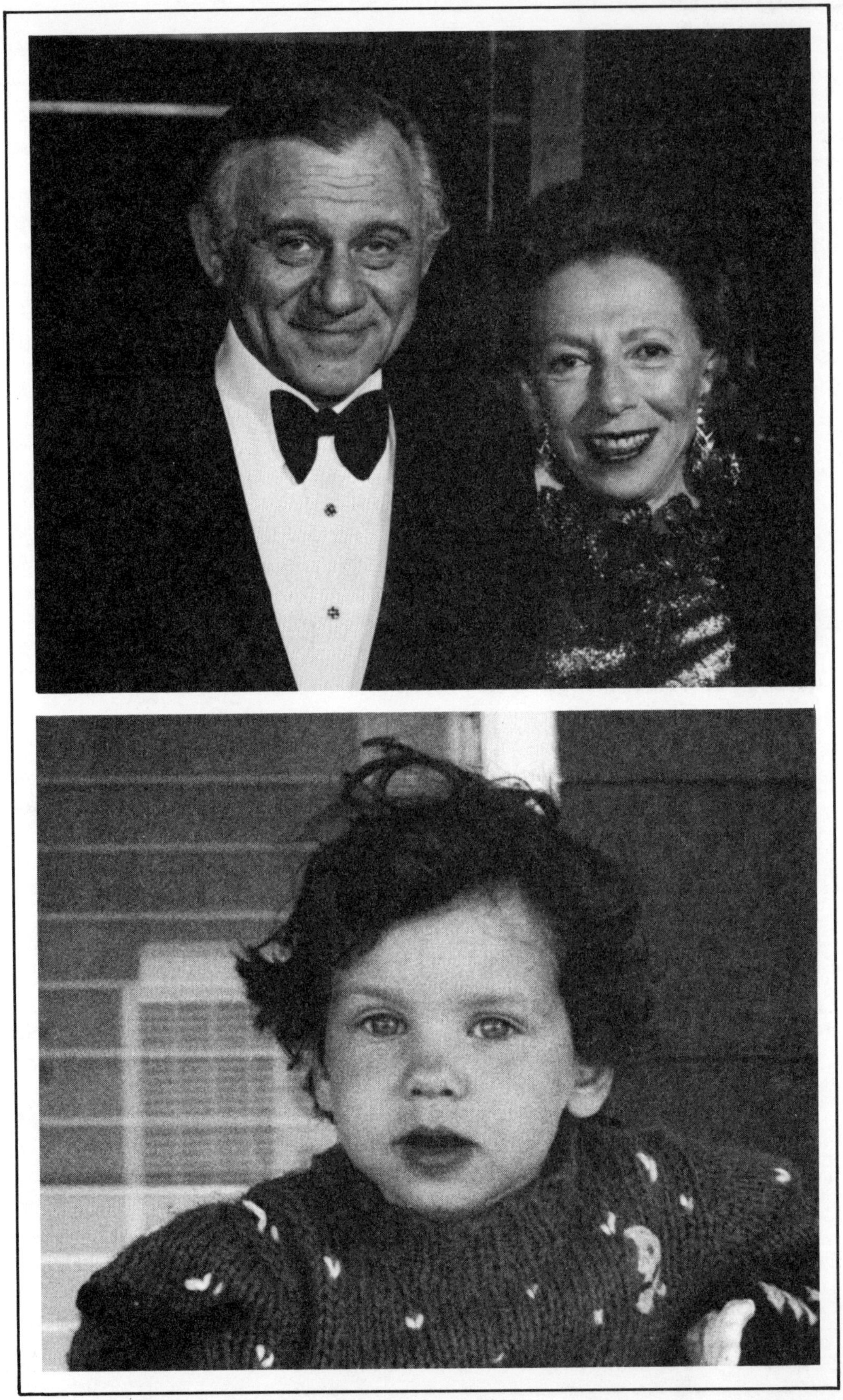

Bernard and Sylvia Green and their granddaughter Lindsay

Sylvia and Bernard Green
New York, New York

Sylvia and Bernard Green were on vacation in Paris when the phone call came telling them that their granddaughter, Lindsay, had Crohn's disease.

Lindsay was just two and a half years old. Since infancy, she had experienced many of the classic signs of IBD: fever, diarrhea, rectal bleeding. When she started talking, she began telling her parents that her tummy hurt, her knees hurt. She was tired, listless, and she had no interest in food. No doctor could find what was wrong.

Frustrated and angry, Bernard Green, a senior partner in a New York City accounting firm, urged his daughter and son-in-law, Lindsay's parents, to keep a diary of her symptoms, *anything* to help doctors reach a diagnosis. Finally, a pediatric gastroenterologist made the diagnosis.

The Greens felt that raising money for research was the best way to help Lindsay and others like her.

"We had to do something." This is the way Bernard Green describes the way he and his wife, Sylvia, felt upon hearing the news. The "something" they agreed to do was raising enough money to fund research in IBD. They felt this was the best way to help Lindsay and others like her. The Greens were no strangers to fund raising, having long been active with the United Fund in their Long Island community, the United Jewish Appeal, and many other philanthropic organizations. Immediately, the Greens and the couple with whom they were vacationing each pledged $10,000 to the research programs of the NFIC. Barely six months later, the total raised by the Greens reached nearly $100,000, enough to sponsor a two-year research project investigating the relationship between nutrition and the use of immunosuppressive drugs in IBD.

Today, at age three and a half, Lindsay's round face betrays the effects of steroid therapy. So far she is growing normally, and doesn't complain often of pain. But her grandfather worries that growing up, as difficult as it is today, will be even more difficult for her. "She will have to live under a cloud until something is discovered," he says.

Because Lindsay, their first grandchild, is so special to them, Sylvia and Bernard Green have already started on their second $100,000.

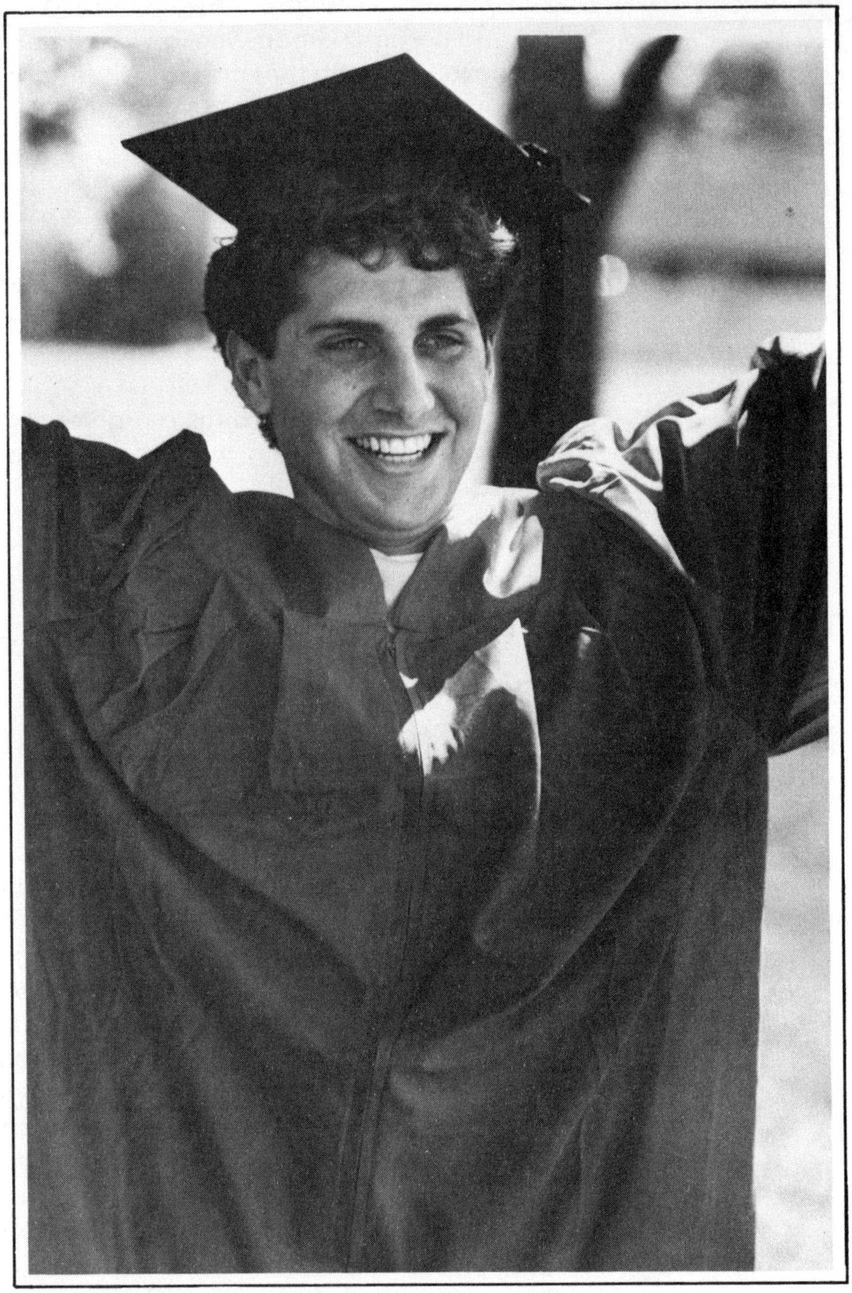

Jimmy Burchfield, Jr.—Photo by Irwin Sterbakov

Jimmy Burchfield, Jr.
Providence, Rhode Island

Jimmy Burchfield, Jr., an athletic, vital young man is the picture of health. Graduated from Boston University and now enrolled in law school, he holds out his strong hand, cups it, points to his palm, and says, "The future is mine, right here." One would never know that Jimmy has had a new, highly complex surgical procedure called the endorectal pull-through. It was this surgery that gave back to Jimmy the control that a ravaging case of ulcerative colitis had taken from him.

"I always knew that I could lick this because I knew surgery was an alternative, but in the beginning I felt surgery was giving up."

His ulcerative colitis was diagnosed in his freshman year of college at a time when he was looking forward to studies, sports, and fun. Jimmy's physician had him experiment with different diets. "My friends were eating pizza and drinking beer, but not me." The disease worsened, his weight dropped from 170 to 102 lbs., and he was put on high doses of steroids. Unfortunately, he had side effects that were at times as distressing as the disease. He felt that he could handle things better emotionally if he kept busy, so he worked weekends while going to school. When that didn't work, he slowed down and decided to take it easy. There was still no improvement. Nothing seemed to work: diets, medication, changing life styles.

Surgery was suggested. Jimmy says, "I always knew that I could lick this because I knew surgery was an alternative, but in the beginning I felt surgery was giving up."

Jimmy's gastroenterologist told him about a new, then still experimental operation. Unlike the standard ileostomy, this procedure, called the endorectal pull-through, does not involve an opening in the abdomen or the wearing of an appliance. Jimmy was well aware of the risks involved, and he knew that the outcome did not have the predictability and reliability of the standard ileostomy. Yet, he says, "I saw it as the best solution to my problem. To me the risks were worth the control I had lost in my life."

Jimmy was determined that his body be in the best shape possible for his surgery. He says, "Working out was the only thing that made me feel better. I ran, used free weights, Nautilus equipment." Jimmy was training for all those years of college sports that he had missed, training for the most important "event" of his life.

He trained in another way, too. Surrounded by his friends and an unusually close family, he worked hard at keeping a positive attitude about the outcome of the surgery. Still, there were difficult times. A week before the operation, he got sick at a family party celebrating his brother's confirmation. He was so upset at ruining the party that he broke down and cried.

A few days later, he had lunch with his physician, who explained to Jimmy that soon the disease would be removed from his body, that there would be only healthy tissue left. Jimmy says that at this point he could visualize his new healthy body and his optimistic spirit returned. He spent the day before his hospital admission with his father; in the morning they went to church. Jimmy entered the hospital on the day of the Boston Marathon. He looked out the window and saw the runners. "A good omen," he thought.

The surgery went fine, but while Jimmy was in the recovery room he had a serious complication. An artery burst, seven pints of blood were lost, and all vital signs stopped. He was rushed back to surgery and spent two days in intensive care.

After the surgeries were completed, he did not have the long physical adjustment most patients are told to expect. He had no pain or cramping, but near normal bowel function. Control was back in Jimmy's life.

It would have been easy for Jimmy to put his past behind him, and to just go on with his life. After all, he was cured. His family could protect him, keeping the intimate details of Jimmy's struggle to themselves.

The Burchfields aren't like that. When Jimmy was first diagnosed, his father said that he would do whatever he could to find a cure. In 1981, working with NFIC's Rhode Island Chapter, Jimmy's father held the first Classic Road Race. Remembering that he himself had never heard of Crohn's disease and ulcerative colitis when his son was diagnosed, he set up a booth and handed out brochures. About three hundred runners participated in that first 8-mile run. Since then the Classic has turned into a world class competition. Last year 150 runners competed, and 15,000 spectators watched.

Jimmy Burchfield, Jr. runs the full eight miles now. He says, "If you really want something, nothing can stop you." He is helping millions of others to regain control over their lives. He has trained well.

Reprinted with permission from The Newsletter, Greater Boston Chapter, NFIC.

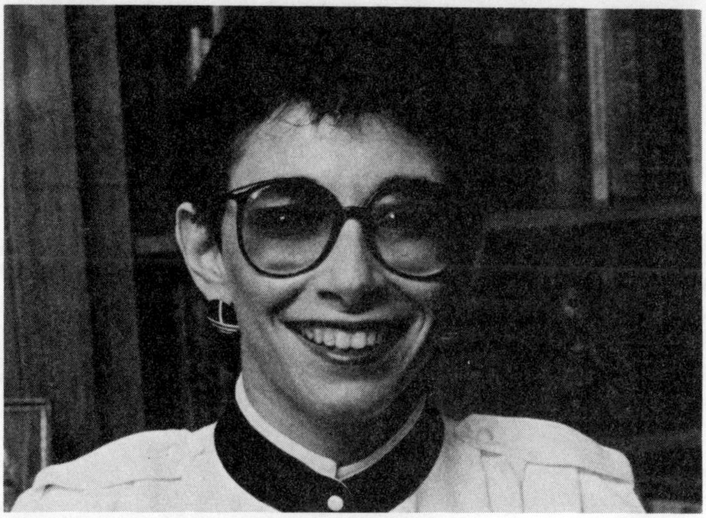

'Pearl's People' No Longer Fear The Worst

For many victims of inflammatory bowel disease, a diagnosis signaled an end for hope. But Pearl Lewis changed all of that.

BY ELLIE FIER
Special To The Baltimore Jewish Times

In a Pikesville home, a small group of people gather to watch a video tape that deals with a special problem they all share. The guests are men, women, and children who are either patients or relatives of patients who suffer a chronic digestive tract disorder called inflamatory bowel disease (IBD); the umbrella term for ulcerative colitis and Crohn's disease. Symptoms can be so debilitating that families have been known to break up because of them.

The matron of this Pikesville home, Pearl Lewis, is herself afflicted. Crohn's disease has caused her nine operations and body altering surgery. (An ileostomy resulted in a reservoir pouch connected to her body which collects body wastes.)

But while Pearl looks fit and keeps active, she can't sit or stand for long periods of time. She can't eat what other people eat, and she suffers a sense of urgency that makes her life revolve around the bathroom.

The people here tonight understand Pearl's problems. Few others do. It's not the kind of sickness one wants to talk about. The pain, embarrassment, fear and worry have become their private burdens — private, that is, until they met Pearl. She organized them into a support group so that now they share their feelings, listen to each other's complaints, and applaud each other's triumphs. The tape, informative and reassuring, helps explain the nature of their disease while it dispells shame and fosters hope. So does Pearl Lewis.

Nineteen-year old Janie Rosenwald is about to undergo surgery.

"I couldn't have done it without her," she says. "Pearl braced my spirits."

Janie, a college theater major, has suffered agonizing bouts with Crohn's disease since she was 10. Last summer, her belly swollen and unable to eat solid food for two months, she lay despondent at home, fed through a tube in her chest.

"I knew just what Janie was feeling," confesses Pearl. "This lovely, talented girl was waiting to die."

Pearl recalls what it was like to be helpless — to be fed, bathed, walked and turned. But, holding Janie's hand, she assured her that she wouldn't die, that she would go through the operation and recover.

"Pearl not only understood my fears," says Janie, "she shared her own feelings with me, described her operations and told me how her life had become more meaningful. I wasn't alone. Plenty of people have the disease. They work, they marry and they live normal lives. I needed to hear that," says Janie.

More than half the population in the United States is affected by digestive diseases, Pearl Lewis points out. Twenty million cases are chronic; 14 million suffer acute episodes, and 100 million others suffer intermittently.

"What's sad," observes Dr. Bob Mathieson, assistant chief of gastroenterology at Union Memorial Hospital, "is that doctors are either not trained, or are unwilling, or have no time to give the emotional support these patients need. They are so scientific that the patient gets lost." So it was with Henrietta Kantor.

At 72, hospitalized three times in three months with Crohn's disease, Mrs. Kantor lost 50 pounds. Not knowing what was happening to her, she feared the worst.

"Pearl taught me how to take care of myself," says Mrs. Kantor. "She gave me courage. She directed me to the right physician and the places where I learned to control my diet. She took my fears away."

Mrs. Kantor is now recovered from surgery and "managing" her ailment. "When I send a greeting card to a member of our support group," she says cheerfully, "I write: 'Dear old Crohnie; We are the lucky ones. We know Pearl.' "

For the past few years Pearl Lewis has been working independently, motivating people to get on with their lives. She encourages those with chronic disorders to take charge of their ailments, to form an alliance with their physicians and learn all they can. "People are suffering needlessly because of ignorance," she declares.

In 1983, Pearl formed the first support group in Baltimore for the families and patients who suffer from ulcerative colitis and Crohn's disease. An ad in the Jewish Times brought 55 people to her home. Today, the newly appointed director of the Baltimore chapter of NFIC (National Foundation of Illetis and Colitis) — it has become a full time job with a small salary — Pearl accounts for more than 600 members. "I wanted to provide education and support, something that didn't exist for these patients before," she says.

"Pearl has done an incredible job of uniting patients with doctors and hospital facilities," affirms Dr. Mathieson. "She's done it single handedly."

According to Dr. Mathieson, the goals of NFIC are ambitious. "Not only does NFIC organize support groups and educational sessions for patients to understand their illness, but raises funds for research. We don't yet know what causes IBD" explains Dr. Mathieson, "but we're learning how to improve the quality of life of those afflicted.

Mayor Schaefer has recognized Pearl and the important role of the non-profit health agency she represents. With the mayor' support, she is forming a coalition of all support groups that deal with any of the chronic diseases. Its purpose, says Pearl, is to provide for those afflicted, the day-to-day coping mechanisms they would not ordinarily receive.

"It's not unusual to see Pearl Lewis at Sinai Hospital these days addressing the health care professionals. Or at Hopkins. Or exchanging ideas on how to help patients at the National Institute of Health. "She is the life line to other patients who haven't yet travelled her road," says one doctor.

Pearl's energy doesn't emanate from a strong physical constitution. She often does not feel well. But at 40, the slim, dark haired mother of six has made a choice: "I could either sit back and be an observer of life, or become a participant." Pearl decided she wouldn't let pain or discomfort deter her, that she had an overriding will to live, and to help others live.

Pearl Lewis—Photo by Craig Terkowitz, *Baltimore Jewish Times*, Copyright 1985

7

Growing Up With IBD

Inflammatory bowel disease affects many young people at a time in their lives when they are trying to achieve some independence and establish their own identities. Having a chronic disease such as Crohn's disease or ulcerative colitis makes it more difficult for young people to develop the skills that are needed to mature and become independent. Gaining self-confidence and adequate social and communication skills can be challenging enough without the disruptive and often difficult tasks associated with managing an illness. The di-

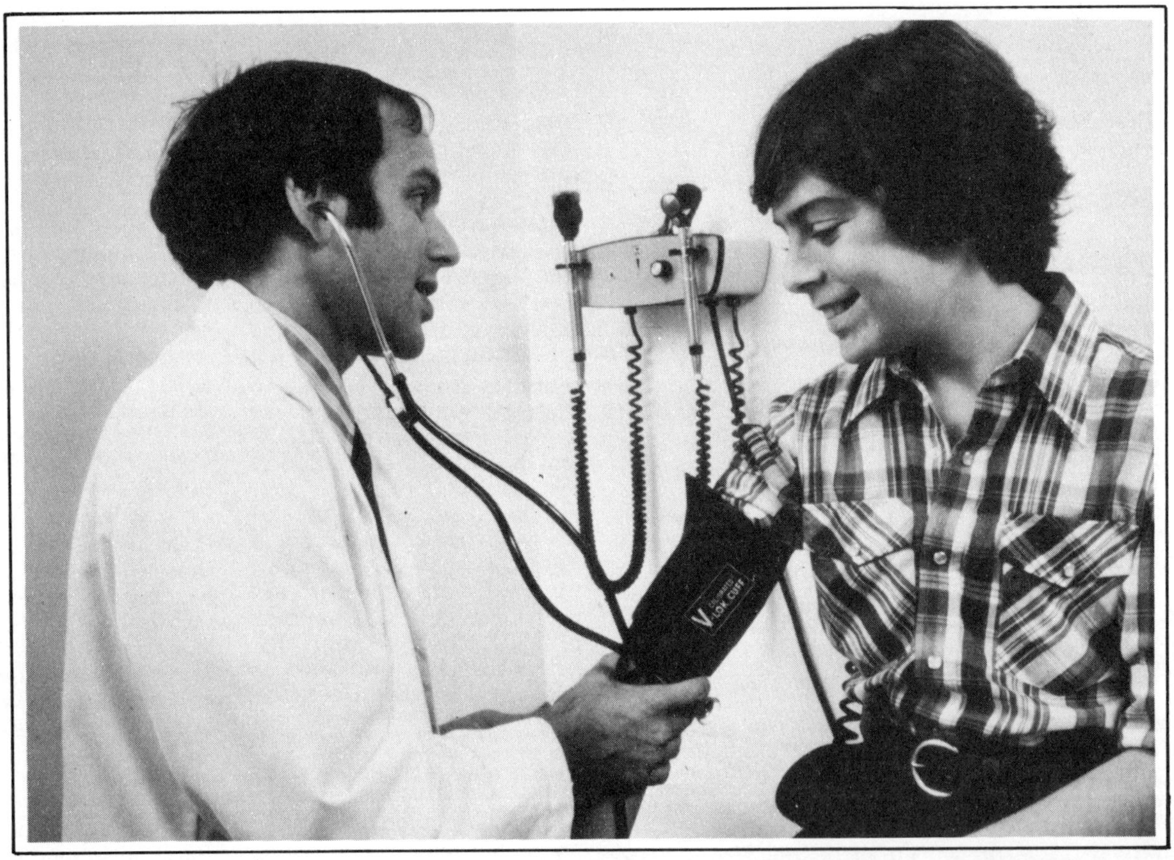

agnosis of a chronic illness can make young people feel different from their peers, diminish their self-confidence and control over their lives, and cause them to feel isolated and unable to convey their thoughts and needs. Health care providers, teachers, family, friends and others can help these young people by being aware of their needs and by being active participants in fostering normal social and school development.

The specific needs of young people with IBD differ with each individual but can be grouped into three areas:

- Obtaining information about their disease and sharing it with others;
- Expressing feelings about IBD and how it affects their lives;
- Taking care of themselves and establishing control in their lives.

Although no one can make the challenges of adapting to a chronic illness go away, we can make adaptation easier and diminish the disruption of the developmental process by recognizing these three areas of need in four environments of the young person: the health care system, the school, the family, and peers.

Sharing Information

Sharing information is a two-way process. The young person needs information from health care providers in order to understand the disease, its diagnosis, and management. The young person then can take this information and share it with family and friends and, as appropriate, with schools and employers. Being able to share information is a positive sign of adjustment in the young person. Sharing information with appropriate persons in authority can help make some environments more hospitable to the young person with IBD.

Talking about IBD can be embarrassing for young people; they may find it extremely difficult to discuss diarrhea and bowel habits openly. If adults associated with these young people can assume a direct, matter-of-fact manner in dealing with these issues, it may ease the sharing of embarrassing information. At the same time, it is necessary to allow young people to set their own limits in relating their knowledge and concerns. Then you can respond to them in a comfortable manner that enhances this communication process.

Negotiating with the School

School nurses and teachers will often be more helpful and understanding if they know about IBD and its symptoms. The doctor could be asked to write a note for school personnel about the disease, or the young person might want to give them this book or NFIC's pamphlet, "A Teacher's Guide to Crohn's Disease and Ulcerative Colitis."

Getting to school and staying a whole day may be a difficult task for the young person with IBD. Attacks of pain and diarrhea may be frequent, and may occur suddenly and without warning. Being able to get to a bathroom quickly is a major concern. Not only is there a fear of having an accident, but the whole subject is one of embarrassment to children and adolescents with IBD. Having a conference with teachers and the school nurse will help them to understand these fears and special needs. Having a prearranged agreement to enable a student to leave the classroom and go to the nearest appropriate bathroom when necessary will go a long way toward making it possible for the person to attend school and not suffer embarrassment.

IBD can cause malnutrition and severe stunting of growth. It is common for young people to feel tired, weak, and just hurt too much to attend school, even when they look well enough. Teachers and school nurses may be more responsive if they understand this. Absence from school is common and clear communication with school personnel can make them more willing to help the student make up work and get homework assignments. If too much time is missed through illness or hospitalization, a homebound teacher may be needed so that the student can keep up with assignments. Occasional hospitalizations make continuing with school work extremely difficult. However, hearing from teachers and classmates can help make young people motivated to return to active school participation.

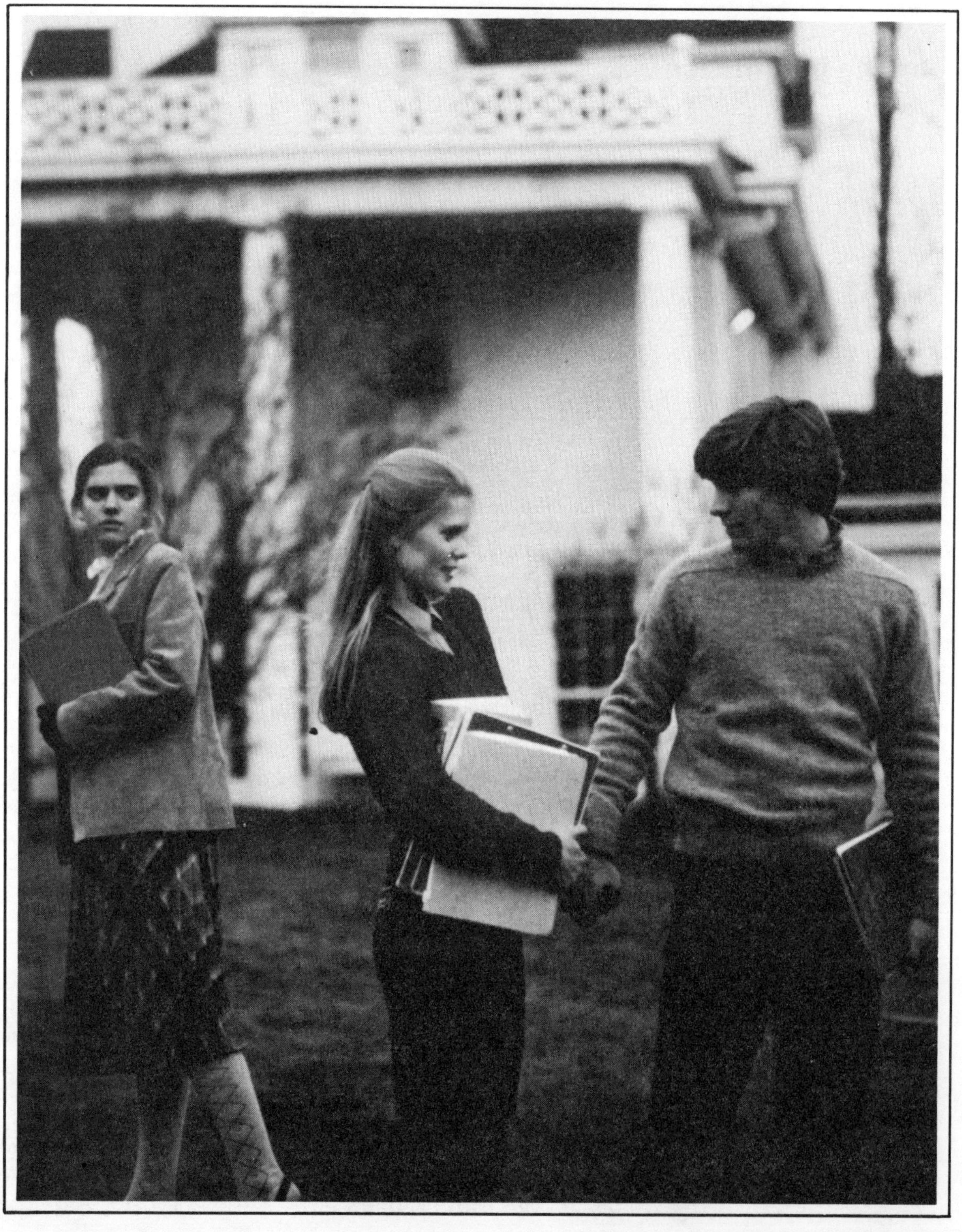

Expressing Feelings

Managing an illness like Crohn's disease or ulcerative colitis creates unique and unpredictable feelings in adolescents and young adults. Chronic disease often leads to feelings of helplessness, anger and depression. There are frustrations with having and accepting a chronic disease, plus the attendant problems of finding bathrooms, missing school and dealing with pain. Young people also worry about not growing and developing at the same rate as their friends. They may feel very different and isolated from their peers. Any and all of these feelings are common and normal.

Many psychologists think that being able to express these feelings helps people to resolve them and to cope better with the illness and the problems of daily living. Those around the person with IBD can be instrumental in encouraging the expression of feelings. Listeners, especially health care providers and families, often try to solve problems for the young person. Listening with the goal of understanding is probably more helpful than trying to jump in and solve problems.

Here are some of the specific behaviors involved in effective interpersonal skills:

- Maintain eye contact.
- Express interest and warmth.
- Allow expression of the person's feelings.
- Allow the person to complete statements.
- Convey empathy and understanding of the person's feelings.
- Do not judge the appropriateness of the person's feeling or minimize the problems.

How do you apply these interpersonal skills to helping a young person who is experiencing anger, anxiety, or fear? It involves five steps:

1. **Establish contact.** Your goal is to establish a relationship of trust in which you convey a feeling of interest, concern, hope, and a non-judgmental attitude.
2. **Discuss the young person's concerns.** Often a simple statement like, "It must be awfully frustrating when your IBD causes you problems at school and you don't seem to be getting any better," gives the young person a chance to express feelings. Ask open-ended questions that require more than a yes or no answer: "How did it go last night," not "What did you tell Bill about your IBD?" Listen, and be non-directive at this point. Let the young person speak. As he/she talks, occasionally paraphrase what feelings and facts are being conveyed: "So the side effects of the prednisone are what's bothering you. You must be wondering if they will *ever* go away."
3. **Discuss alternatives.** "Should you call the doctor and talk about your medications?" Sometimes the young person is just angry about the loss of control; in this case, ask, "What do you think we should do now?"
4. **Provide support.** "I know these are big problems but I think you can manage them. Hang in there!" In some cases, self-disclosure is very effective in providing support: "When I was a teenager I had to wear a cast for a year. I thought I looked like a large watermelon with legs," or even, "I'm upset *too*

about what you're going through." If you're not getting anywhere, share your frustation: "I'm not sure we're getting very far right now—where would you like to go from here?" Remember that the inflection and intensity of your voice, facial expressions, and body language need to match the words you are saying.

5. **Bring about closure.** Agree on a course of action, possibly including talking with someone else. Restate your support, and always conclude on a note of hope: "OK, you're already looking better just talking about this."

Thus, in the course of five to ten minutes, you can greatly assist the young person to regain a sense of hope and self-confidence.

Promoting Self Care and Self Control

A chronic illness can sometimes thwart the normal development of self control and independence. Promoting self care and active involvement in the normal activities of daily living can help ease this impact.

Sometimes when people are ill they expect their doctors and nurses to make them well. They do not expect to have to do much in order to get well. As you probably know by now, this is not the case with Crohn's disease or ulcerative colitis. A person with IBD needs to work *with* the doctor to keep the disease under control.

The doctor needs the young person with IBD to be able to do several things:

- Take medication and report side effects.
- Solve problems that might interfere with taking medication or following dietary recommendations.
- Keep track of symptoms and report them to their doctor.

Any person with IBD needs to be responsible for his/her own medications. Occasionally people do not take the medication their doctors have prescribed. No one is positive why this happens, but there are probably different reasons for different people. For some people keeping track of taking the medications is a "hassle." One kind of hassle is a complex schedule. Several things can help young people with taking medications: keeping a medication calendar; taking medications at the same time every day; and taking medications at the same time as another activity that they do every day like brushing their teeth or eating meals. Sometimes young people or their parents may need to negotiate with the school to allow for the taking of medications during the day.

Certain IBD medications, such as cortisone-like drugs, can cause troublesome side effects. These include excessive weight gain, a puffy face, worsening of acne, and moodiness. These can cause serious problems for a young person who is concerned with physical attractiveness and fitting in with peers. Providing information about the medications and their side effects (including that the side effects are temporary and will diminish as the dose is lowered) may help. Expressing feelings about the side effects may also help make them more tolerable. If scheduling or side effects are a problem, perhaps the schedule or medication dosage can be negotiated with the doctor.

Other areas of concern to the teenager are diet and physical activity. In general, patients with IBD are encouraged to eat a regular diet and participate in sports and physical activity as much as possible. There will be times when this is not possible, and specific restrictions will be needed. An understanding teacher who will encourage participation with rest periods as needed can help the person set his/her own limits and cope better with the disease.

Most of the time, young people are encouraged to eat a well balanced diet to maintain their growth. However, there are times when symptoms are worse and a special or limited diet may be needed. Eating in the school cafeteria may be hard under these circumstances, but food can be brought from home to supply the appropriate nutrients.

Many teenagers struggle with their parents to be allowed to have more freedom, and to do things on their own. Some people with IBD report that after they have been sick, they feel like their parents take more control over them and they lose their independence. When this happens, the teenager and the parents may become angry with each other and with the disease. If young people with IBD are having these problems, some understanding between them and their parents will help.

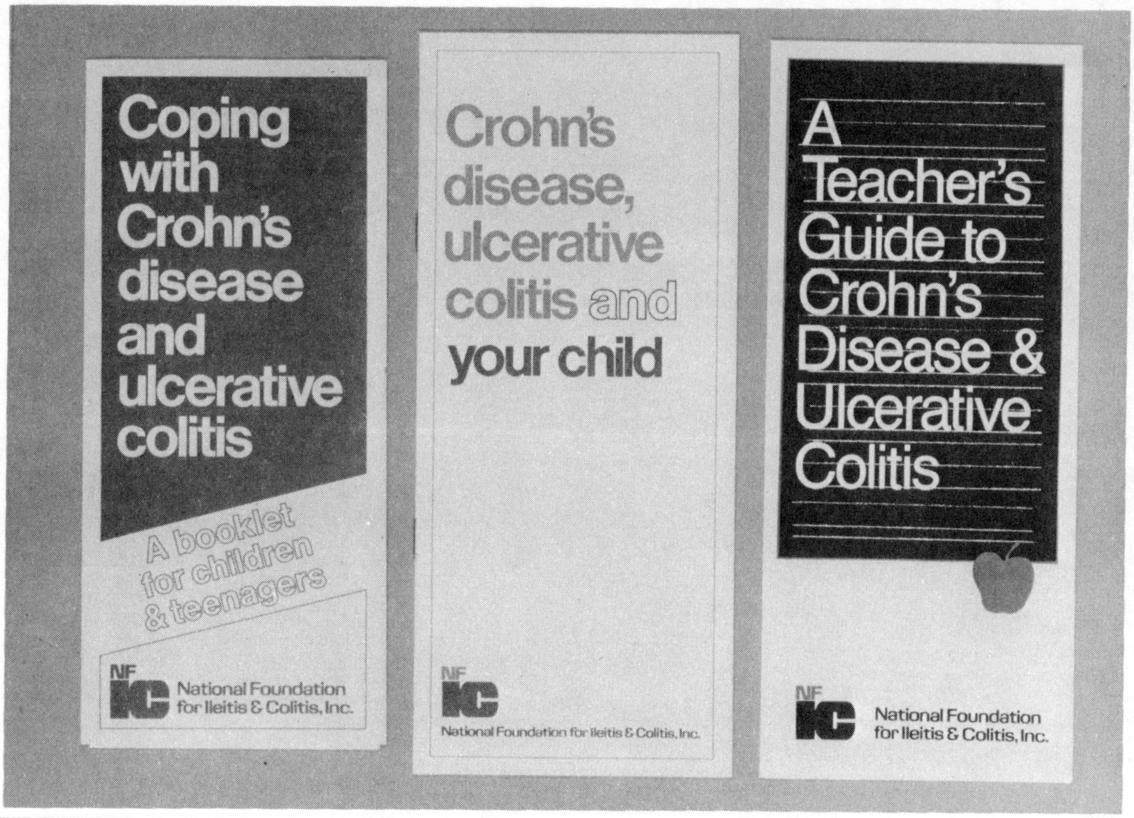

Young people might need to understand that when they are sick their parents are very concerned and want to take care of them. However, being taken care of can cause conflicting feelings in adolescents who are striving for independence. The same attention parents gave them when they were feeling sick might be too much attention when they are feeling well.

Parents might need to understand that being independent and trying new things is a natural and positive part of being an adult. They also need to know that young people feel better about themselves when they make their own decisions. They can find ways to show their children that they love them without overprotecting them. Young people might want to tell their parents how they *can* help. In this way, they show their parents that they are in control of the situation and also let them know that they appreciate the help.

Overall, it is important to remember that having a chronic illness makes young people feel as if they are losing some control over their lives. These guidelines may help people with IBD get through these rough times:

Young people should:

- Let their family, friends or doctor know when they are feeling "out of control" or when they just need to talk.
- Take control over things they can control—for example, taking medicine and talking with the doctor by themselves.
- Keep in contact with friends.
- Remember that things will change. Just because young people may be dependent when they are sick does not mean they cannot be independent when they are well.

8 How To Communicate With Your Doctor

Introduction

Crohn's disease and ulcerative colitis are chronic illnesses that cause unexpected disruptions in daily living. The emotional and physical impact of these illnesses can be debilitating. It is extremely important that you have access to an understanding physician who provides the best medical treatment in a supportive and helpful manner.

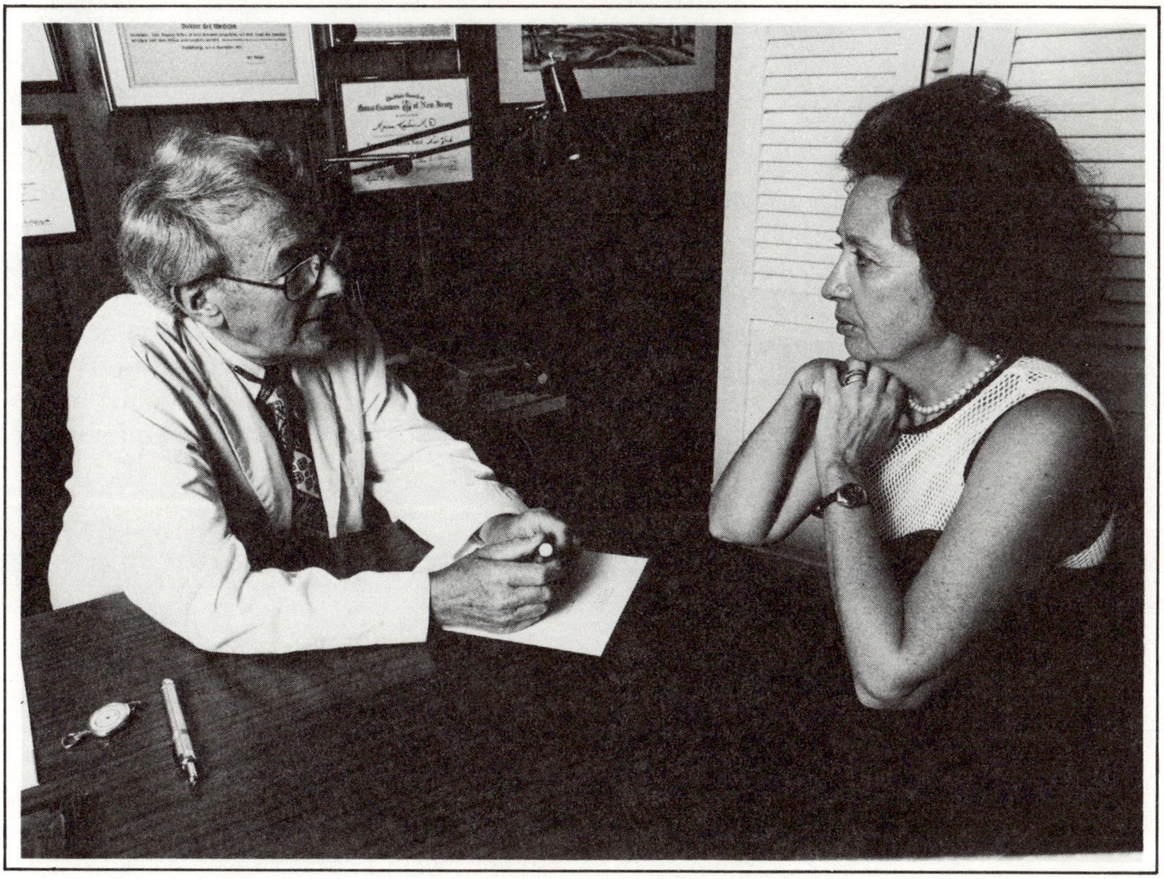

The interaction between patient and physician may have an important bearing on the way in which a person copes with chronic illness. A recent study in the *Annals of Internal Medicine* found that people with chronic illnesses who took a more active role in communicating with their physicians coped better with their disease on a daily basis.

Those who became more assertive in seeking information had a greater impact on decisions that influenced their health and medical treatment. On the other hand, patients who remained relatively uninformed and did not take an active role in their care were less prepared to integrate treatment programs into workable daily routines that could help them cope with their illnesses.

It may be difficult for the person with IBD to find a physician who has the medical approach and personality suited to a relationship that may last for many years.

People vary in personality and needs; this is also true when they become patients. Some deny illness, avoid office visits, and expect physicians to do only what is minimally required to keep them well. Others require frequent reassurance on the telephone, numerous office visits, and need a physician who is available at all times to answer questions. Some people respond to an intellectual, scholarly approach, while others need a more personal, caring approach. Happily, most people fall somewhere between these extremes. It may be difficult for the person with IBD to find a physician who has the medical approach and personality suited to a relationship that may last for many years. Mutual trust is a major component of this relationship: for the patient, trust that the physician is competent and compassionate; for the physician, trust that the patient will be honest and forthright and will become a true partner in the treatment process.

What to Expect of Your Physician

Your physician should be accessible to you. You should be able to reach him/her or an associate during the day, at night, on weekends, and especially in case of an emergency. When you visit the office, you should expect knowledgeable treatment of your illness. He or she should be sensitive to your emotional and physical well-being and should be willing to talk frankly about the outlook for the future and the goals you will set together.

Who should be your physician? There are two possibilities. Your first choice would be a board certified gastroenterologist (or pediatric gastroenterologist) with a specific interest in inflammatory bowel disease. Being board certified means that your physician has spent the required number of years in a recognized and approved training program in internal medicine and gastroenterology (usually 4 to 5 years), and has passed examinations given by the American Board of Gastroenterology. Your local NFIC chapter and the National Office have referral lists of certified gastroenterologists in your area. You can also call the state or county medical society and ask for the names of qualified physicians who have special training or who have indicated a strong interest in the management of inflammatory bowel disease. Each public library has a directory of licensed physicians listed by specialty.

A second choice is an internist or family practice physician who is experienced in treating people with IBD. Many physicians with these credentials can manage IBD problems. If and when difficulties arise in treatment, these physicians can obtain advice from consulting gastroenterologists or surgeons who specialize in IBD.

Many physicians display their diplomas in their offices. If you do not see them, you have the right to ask where your physician attended medical school and completed internship and residency, and whether he or she is board certified in gastroenterology.

Your physician's office should have a comfortable, well-ventilated waiting room, clean, private examining rooms, and accessible bathrooms. The office staff should be courteous, sensitive, and understanding. When discussing medical or financial matters, they should talk quietly to insure privacy. They should address you in a way that you find comfortable. If you have strong feelings about the way you are addressed by staff or physician, you have every right to say so. If you sense a recurring problem in any area of the office, it is appropriate to tell your physician about it.

Your physician should be on time for your appointments. This is often difficult since no physician refuses an urgent telephone call from a patient, from a colleague requiring an immediate advice, or a hospital nurse reporting a change in the condition of a patient. If you are the person who is waiting, try to understand the possible reasons for these interruptions. At another time, it could be you.

After being examined, you should have the opportunity to discuss your care with the physician in the consulting room with the door closed and no telephone interruptions. This need not take place after every visit, but should be available when there are important issues that must be discussed.

What Your Physician Expects of You

In this partnership of mutual trust, you should not expect an immediate response from your physician for a routine problem. You should understand that physicians are frequently too busy, and must take care of emergency problems first, urgent cases second, and routine problems last. If you require an immediate response, you should state this clearly. If the response is not needed until the end of the day or the next day, you should make that clear as well. Inform the office or answering service about what is the best time for the physician to return the call, and make sure that no one is using the phone at that time. Telephone calls on weekends and in the evenings are for urgent and emergency problems *only*! In these situations, you may reach an associate of the physician who is on call and does not know the details of your medical problem. If the communication can wait until the next day, you may be better off waiting to reach your own doctor.

Renewals of medication should be requested with time to spare. If renewal of medication is complex, it is a good idea to send a note to the physician outlining the requirements. This is especially important if you are planning to be away for a prolonged interval.

Whether you are telephoning your physician or visiting the office, you should have a very clear and concise list of questions to ask. Very long lists are not appropriate. Physicians are people too, and may become weary or impatient when faced with exhausting questions with each visit or phone call. Decide what is important *before* contacting your physician.

Taking the time to get to know and respect the office staff can be a great help to you when you are trying to reach your doctor.

You should also inform your physician which member of your family should be kept informed about your progress. This can be a parent, spouse, or any other person you wish. The physician should not respond to requests for information from a family member unless you have given permission for him/her to disclose this information. It is sometimes advisable for this family member to accompany you to medical visits, since he or she can work with you and your physician in reaching important decisions about diagnostic procedures, hospitalization, or surgery.

While in your doctor's office, be aware that the doctor's staff is often overworked and may be dealing with urgent situations. Nurses and secretaries may conceal the fact that there are serious problems that have them very worried. If the office staff appears to be under pressure, hold your routine concerns until a later time. Taking the time to get to know and respect the office staff can be a great help to you when you are trying to reach your doctor.

Choosing a Surgeon

When necessary, your primary physician will call in a surgeon for a consultation. Personality and compatibility are important qualities in a surgeon, but they are not nearly as important as his/her surgical skill. The surgeon of your choice should be someone with a combination of experience and common sense. Important details include academic credentials, experience in performing surgery in IBD, and the number of similar operations he or she has performed in the preceding year.

There are many questions you need to ask about the surgery itself. First, who will be actually performing the surgery: this surgeon, an associate, or a surgical resident? At some large teaching institutions, physicians delegate some of the surgical procedures to senior resident surgeons in training. These surgeons often have five or more years of experience and are highly qualified. You should also ask who will be giving your postoperative care, both in the hospital and afterward. This is particularly important if a newer operaton such as an ileoanal anastomosis or a continent ileostomy is being considered.

When the decision to operate has been reached, the surgeon should discuss the major potential complications of the surgery well in advance of the date of your operation. If the surgeon does not initiate this discussion, you should feel free to ask any of the questions you need answered. Before surgery, you will be asked to sign a consent form, a medical legal document certifying that you understand the nature of the operation and its possible complications. Make sure that you are an informed patient.

Finally, you should be told the cost of the procedure and follow-up care. If there are questions about your insurance coverage, these should be discussed with your surgeon or the office staff. Any request for a reduced fee, for whatever reason, should be made in advance.

When to Get a Consultation

Even in the best patient-doctor relationship, there may be a need for a second opinion in the form of a consultation with a gastroenterologist or surgeon. There are many valid reasons for this. There may be a major deterioration in the pattern of your illness, or your condition may not be responding to current medical treatment. As a result, your physician may be ready to suggest a major change in therapy, such as the introduction of a new medication, hyperalimentation, hospitalization, or surgery.

Your physician may be the one to suggest a consultation. However, a good doctor should never feel hurt or threatened if you request a consultation. Such a request may even increase the sense of shared responsibility between doctor and patient. It is far better to discuss the request for a second opinion with your physician rather than to obtain a consultation without his or her knowledge. Your physician may then sense a lack of trust which may influence your relationship from that point on.

Regardless of who initiates the request for a consultation, your physician should then give you the names of reliable physicians whom you may consult. Your physician should also make your records and x-rays available and should make the initial telephone call or write a letter to the consultant to familiarize him/her with your case. Whenever possible, hand carry as much information to the consultant as possible. This includes your x-ray folder, which may be delayed or even lost if mailed. Since you are the legal "owner" of the information contained in your office records and x-rays, you will need to sign a release form to legalize the transfer of information (See Chapter 15).

When you see the consultant, be prepared to present your medical history, including the time of onset, pattern of illness, dates of admissions to hospitals, surgical procedures, types of medications and dosages. This information should be given in chronological order. It is frequently helpful to bring a concise written history containing this information in outline form. Be clear, logical, and specific about why you are seeking the consultation. You should receive a full physical examination and should have enough time in the consultation room so that all your questions are answered.

A good doctor should never feel hurt or threatened if you request a consultation.

Following the visit, a consulting physician should write a letter to your physician summarizing his/her findings and recommendations. You should then call or see your physician to discuss the recommendations. If the consultant has agreed with the plans initially outlined by your physician, you and your physician should be reassured. If there are differences, further discussion and additional input from other physicians may be required to chart an appropriate course for your treatments.

Editors' Note

Sometimes, even under the best of circumstances, you may become dissatisfied with the care you are receiving from your physician. If this happens, you have every right to find another physician whose approach may be better suited to your needs. IBD is a frustrating illness for both patient and physician, and a change of physician may be helpful. NFIC chapters have lists of board certified gastroenterologists and other specialists in their geographic areas.

Good Medical Care When You Can't Afford It

If your medical insurance coverage has lapsed at the time of a flare-up or if you have no coverage for office visits, consider visiting the gastroenterology clinic at a major medical center. As a general rule, these clinics are staffed by gastrointestinal residents under the supervision of a senior gastroenterologist. The chances are that you will be seen by a physician who is already qualified in internal medicine and is working toward certification in gastroenterology. Your x-rays will be performed by a radiology resident, supervised by an attending radiologist, and such procedures as endoscopy will be performed under the supervision of a senior physician. The clinic physician will take a history and perform a physical examination, and you will be followed regularly at fees which are estimated according to your ability to pay. There are also a few private clinics that are willing to perform a similar service. The NFIC National Office can provide you with a list of clinics in your geographical area.

In a gastroenterology clinic at a major medical center, you will be followed regularly at fees which are estimated according to your ability to pay.

Some private physicians also treat patients at reduced rates. If the doctor agrees, be honest about the limitations of your financial resources. Make an effort to pay something every month, even if it is a small amount, to let the physician know that you have appreciated this courtesy to you. You might even consider volunteering to be part of a research project at a major teaching institution, such as those testing new medications. At these centers, all research projects are carefully scrutinized by a Human Subjects Committee and are carefully monitored under the federal Privacy Act. If you are a good candidate for a particular project, you will be assured of good follow-up care on a regular basis by qualified physicians.

Editors' Note

If you are unable to pay anything for medical office visits yet are not eligible for Medicaid in your state, you may still be eligible for free care in hospital out-patient clinics under the Hill-Burton Act.

In 1946 Congress passed a law which gave hospitals and other health facilities money for construction and modernization. In return, the facilities which received these Hill-Burton funds agreed to provide a reasonable volume of services to persons unable to pay, and to make their services available to all persons residing in the facility's area. The Department of Health and Human Services (DHHS) is responsible for the administration of this program.

Write your Department of Health and Human Services (DHHS) Regional Office or call the following toll-free number:

1-800-638-0742

for Maryland Residents: 1-800-492-0359

Danger Signals: When to Call Your Doctor

It is useful to separate telephone calls to your physician into three categories: routine, urgent and emergency. Your doctor should always tell you when you may place routine calls to the office, for example, to obtain the results of blood and laboratory tests or to report any changes in your symptoms. Your doctor will undoubtedly want to note the nature of your call on your chart, so it is important to call him or her at a time when the chart is available.

An urgent call is one which is important but not an emergency. An urgent call should be returned by your doctor during the same day. A reason for an urgent call might be the sudden appearance of a rash on your body. A rash might indicate an allergic reaction to a medication or even a new symptom of the illness itself, such as erythema nodosum (painful, tender bumps on your legs which often indicate the start of a flare-up). Other urgent symptoms include swelling of the joints, a persistent low grade fever, or the appearance of a small amount of blood in your stool. When you call your doctor's office with an urgent call, be prepared to be as specific as possible with the office staff. You have the right to ask when you can expect a call back. Be sure to stay off the telephone if you are expecting a return call.

An emergency phone call is justified by an acute, dramatic change in your illness. These changes include:

- a sudden high fever which might be accompanied by shaking chills;
- a sudden weight loss of over five pounds in a few days;
- the onset of significant or new rectal bleeding;
- any severe abdominal pain that persists for longer than an hour;
- persistent vomiting accompanied by cessation of bowel movements;
- a drastic change in bowel movements without passing gas.

It is essential that you convey the emergent nature of your call to the office staff. Your doctor should speak to you at once if he/she is there, or by return phone call.

If you are the type of person who can effectively determine the routine, urgent or emergency nature of your call, you will greatly enhance your relationship with your doctor and the office staff.

Summary

The "perfect" relationship between the person with IBD and the physician may not be possible in today's world. But the responsibility for continued good management of any chronic illness rests with both parties, and succeeds most often when there is a partnership of mutual trust.

9 How To Eat When You Have IBD

The importance of nutrition in maintaining good health is a well-recognized concept of our time. Meeting nutritional needs is necessary for everyone, but is especially important for people with inflammatory bowel disease for at least three reasons. First, medications such as corticosteroids are more effective when your nutritional state is not severely depleted. Second, when intestinal losses of nutrients occur in IBD, they must be compensated for by increasing the amount of food taken in. Third, the slowing of growth which occurs in some children and teenagers with IBD often responds dramatically when caloric and protein intake is increased. Being able to eat sufficient quantities of food is often very difficult when gastrointestinal symptoms are active. In this chapter, we present several approaches that have been helpful in maximizing nutrient intake in IBD.

Facts and Fallacies About Nutrition in IBD

All too often, nutritional counseling for people with IBD sets goals which merely satisfy the nutritional requirements of the healthy population. These recommendations, based upon Recommended Daily Allowances (RDA), may not supply sufficient calories for a person with IBD. For example, the amounts of nutrients, especially calories, protein, and some vitamins and minerals, increase from childhood through puberty and then increase again in adulthood. These general recommendations must be increased even further if an individual has excessive losses of fat, protein, iron, calcium, zinc and other nutrients, or must replenish body stores depleted by chronic undernutrition. The average recommended amount for calories and protein appears in the chart below.

Recommended Daily Allowances*

		Average Daily Carolic Intake (kilocalories)	Average Daily Protein Intake (grams)
Children	(7-10 yrs)	2400	34
Males	(11-14 yrs)	2700	45
	(15-18 yrs)	2800	56
	(19-22 yrs)	2900	56
	(23-50 yrs)	2700	56
	(51-75 yrs)	2400	56
Females	(11-14 yrs)	2200	46
	(15-18 yrs)	2100	46
	(19-22 yrs)	2100	44
	(23-50 yrs)	2000	44
	(51-75 yrs)	1800	44

*Food and Nutrition Board, National Academy of Sciences (1980)

Usually, the nutritional needs of the person with IBD can be met by food alone, together with a well-formulated multivitamin preparation and, if needed, an iron supplement. It is important to recognize that it is the *total daily intake* of calories, protein and other nutrients that is important, not the number of times you eat each day. You may feel more comfortable eating three smaller meals and two or three snacks than the usual three regular meals per day.

Some foods that we consider to be "junk food" often have substantial nutritional value. A slice of pizza provides protein, calcium and vitamin D from the cheese and vitamins A and C from the tomato sauce. Similarly, the hamburgers and cheeseburgers at fast-food chains provide plenty of protein in addition to calories. While foods like these contain more fat and salt than is prudent on a long-term basis, the calories and protein they provide during the growing period can help to maintain normal gains in height and weight for young people with IBD.

Milk products like cheese, milk shakes, and ice cream are an excellent source of calories and protein and should *not* be avoided simply because a child or adult has IBD. In some people, milk sugar (lactose) may cause bloating or diarrhea (lactase deficiency), but the discomfort is usually temporary and can be alleviated with the use of a commercially prepared enzyme (see below). There is no evidence to suggest that these products will aggravate IBD.

Some people with IBD limit their intake of food during daytime hours in order to prevent cramping, trips to the bathroom, or accidents at work or school. Unfortunately, this practice can greatly reduce the number of calories consumed each day. If the physician is made aware of this situation, specific medications can be prescribed and arrangements made with employers or teachers. NFIC's pamphlet for teachers can be helpful in explaining the special needs of children with IBD while they are at school.

At times, the symptoms of IBD can prevent you from eating enough to satisfy nutritional requirements. This can happen when there is narrowing of the bowel or continuous diarrhea. When eating is difficult under these circumstances, liquid formula supplements may be recommended to provide additional nutrients. Many products are now available in a range of flavors and prices. Your doctor may recommend a specific liquid formula when a higher protein content or lower residue diet is necessary. A list of these products is presented in the following chapter.

How to Decrease Intestinal Cramping Associated with Eating

When IBD is active, it is not unusual for eating to cause cramping and intestinal discomfort. This is especially true when the small intestine is involved. Since there are several reasons why this occurs, it is important to observe any association between specific foods or types of foods and the onset of gastrointestinal symptoms. Any of the following foods can cause discomfort:

- **Milk and milk products.** Lactase is an enzyme in the small intestine which breaks down lactose, the sugar found in dairy products. If lactase levels are low, symptoms of bloating, gas and/or diarrhea usually occur 30 to 90 minutes after drinking milk or eating large amounts of cheese or ice cream. (Some dairy products, like butter and yogurt, cause few problems.) Using non-diary (milk substitute) products or adding commercially available lactase to milk for 24-48 hours before drinking will alleviate these symptoms. Recently, predigested milk has become available in grocery stores.

- **High fiber foods.** This category includes foods such as seeds, nuts, popcorn, corn and certain Chinese vegetables. These foods may produce cramping when there is narrowing of the bowel. When this occurs early in the course of the disease, it is often a temporary problem caused by edema or swelling of the bowel wall. When this happens later in the course of illness, it may indicate scarring (stenosis) of the intestine. High fiber foods also contribute to diarrhea (greater stool volume) because they are incompletely digested by the small intestine. Once fiber enters the large intestine, it stimulates contractions, especially when the colon is involved with either Crohn's colitis or ulcerative colitis. This is the reason for using "low residue foods" such as broths, gelatin, poultry without skins, potatoes without skins, rolls, noodles, rice, eggs, and fish. High fiber foods may also contribute to diarrhea by causing mechanical irritation if the colon is severely inflamed. A more complete discussion of this topic can be found in the following chapter.

- **Fried or greasy foods.** This category includes pork products, butter, margarine, cream sauces, etc. These foods may also cause gas and diarrhea if absorption of fat is incomplete. Fat absorption is reduced most often after removal of large amounts of small bowel, especially ileum. One way to overcome these symptoms is to decrease the amount of fat in the diet. Another way is to use an easily absorbable fat supplement, such as MCT oil, in cooking and salad dressings.

- **Large meals.** Many people with IBD find that frequent (perhaps five) small meals produce fewer symptoms than the customary three large meals per day. From a nutritional viewpoint, what matters most is the total amount of calories, protein, and calcium consumed on a daily basis. Despite attention to all of these factors, intestinal discomfort may continue to recur with eating. If this happens, an adjustment in medication may help alleviate the symptoms. Corticosteroid medications such as prednisone may significantly decrease intestinal inflammation and allow the bowel to be more normal in size and function. Other medications (such as antispasmodics and antidiarrheal medications) decrease spasms and diarrhea. When taken 15-20 minutes before eating, these medications prevent symptoms which interrupt meals and encourage greater intake of food. They are most helpful in mild disease and must be used with caution, if at all, in severely active disease (see Chapter 3).

Improving Nutrition when Eating Fails

Sometimes, despite continued attempts at eating, nutritional status deteriorates in IBD. Weight loss may persist and body stores of muscle, fat, and protein diminish. In children and teenagers, the growth rate may slow to below normal. Faced with problems such as these, the physician may adjust the medication schedule or think more seriously about the need for surgery.

In some circumstances, nutritional support can be enhanced by alternative means. One method involves the infusion of liquid formulas directly into the stomach or small bowel through a small, soft feeding tube. Usually, the tube is inserted into the nostril and passed into the stomach each night. It is removed in the morning so that the person can go to school or work. If hospitalization is required, the infusion may continue on a 24-hour basis. This approach has been used successfully to control inflammation and to improve growth in children either alone or in combination with the intake of food during the day. As an alternative, some physicians have used night-time gastrostomy feedings. A gastrostomy is a surgically-made opening through the abdominal wall directly into the stomach, through which the feeding tube is passed. The obvious advantage of this type of feeding is that it is not necessary to pass a tube through the nose each night.

When tube feeding is required, the composition of the liquid formula and the amount infused depend upon the needs of the individual. The short-term results (4-6 weeks) with nasogastric infusion are usually good, indicating improvement in disease activity and growth. Understandably, the acceptance of tube feeding varies and may be higher in children than in late adolescents and adults.

A second method of supplying nutrient requirements is by vein (intravenous route). This approach bypasses the intestine altogether and "rests" the bowel by decreasing the work of digestion and intestinal blood flow. This method was called intravenous "hyperalimentation" in the past, but is now known as total parenteral nutrition (TPN).

TPN can be used temporarily in the hospital or adapted for on-going use at home. Usually the intravenous administration continues during the night but is stopped in the morning so that the person can go to school or work. TPN is expensive, requires a training program in the hospital and has potentially serious complications. It is therefore recommended only in selected situations, such as preparing malnourished patients for surgery, healing severe perianal inflammation or fistulous disease, or reversing growth failure unresponsive to oral nutrition. The technique should be supervised only by a medical team familiar with its management. Currently, this requires a group effort consisting of physician, nurse, nutritionist, and pharmacist.

Many approaches are available to maintain or improve nutritional status of the person with IBD. The easiest and safest methods should be used whenever possible, with the more invasive approaches reserved for special circumstances. Good nutrition depends upon a continuing dialogue between the person with IBD, the gastroenterologist, and the nutritionist or dietitian.

10

A Guide To Food Sources Of Essential Nutrients

Nutrition is an environmental factor which continually affects health and disease. It is important to remember that as far as we know, no food causes IBD, and that dietary modification can actually help reduce disease symptoms and replace lost nutrients. Once IBD is in remission, eating habits can often return to normal. While the health team that cares for you will be the best guide to developing your specific dietary plan, we present the following information to help you choose foods and supplements to carry out that plan.

It is important to remember that as far as we know, no food causes IBD, and that dietary modification can actually help reduce disease symptoms and replace lost nutrients.

Basic Nutritional Requirements

The body makes thousands of different substances daily, but the "essential nutrients" it cannot produce must be provided by the food we eat. These nutrients are made from 25 chemical elements, 11 of which—carbon, hydrogen, oxygen, nitrogen, phosphorus, calcium, sulfur, sodium, potassium, magnesium and chloride—make up 99 percent of the human body. These elements are the building blocks of proteins, fats, carbohydrates, vitamins, water and nucleic acids. They form our bones and teeth and are essential parts of all cells and body fluids. The remaining 1 percent of the body consists of the trace elements, such as zinc, which are no less essential.

Nutritional requirements for the general population have been established by the Food and Nutrition Board of the National Research Council. This board has supplied information on what is termed the Recommended Daily Allowance (RDA) of nutrients. The RDA's are the "levels of intake of essential nutrients considered to be adequate to meet the known nutritional needs of practically all healthy persons."

RDA's are met when one eats a specified number of servings from each of the *Basic Four Food Groups:*

- fruit and vegetables–4 servings
- grain and cereal–4 servings
- dairy–2 to 4 servings
- meat and meat substitutes–2 servings.

Although RDA's are not specified for a particular individual or disease, they are useful as a starting point in planning modifications for patients with IBD. Modifications in diet are often required to lessen the symptoms of IBD, to meet the RDA's for specific nutrients, and to exceed the RDA's whenever necessary in order to correct nutritional deficiencies.

I. Dietary Modification in IBD

Nutritional deficiency in IBD may occur for the following reasons:

- Decreased food intake caused by symptoms or side effects of medications such as sulfasalazine.
- Decreased absorption of food from the small intestine caused by inflammation or the side effects of medications.
- Increased losses of protein or other substances that leak into the bowel lumen from diseased areas.

It is particularly important to be aware of drug-nutrient interactions. Sulfasalazine interferes with the absorption of folic acid, one of the B vitamins. High-dose daily corticosteroids can decrease intestinal absorption of calcium and phosphorus, increase urinary losses of vitamin C, calcium, potassium, zinc, and nitrogen, and cause excessive breakdown of protein. Steroids also cause fluid retention, an effect that can be counteracted by eating a diet lower in salt. A third important medication that may affect nutrients is cholestyramine (Questran) which is sometimes helpful in controlling diarrhea caused by the presence of unabsorbed bile salts in the colon. (Bile salts are normally absorbed in the healthy ileum and recycled by the body.) Unfortunately, cholestyramine may also cause poor absorption of the fat soluble vitamins (A, D, E, and K) as well as folic acid, vitamin B-12, calcium, and iron. Awareness of these drug-nutrient interactions and increased intake of the nutrients affected can help prevent deficiencies.

The diets described below may be encountered at one time or another during the course of your treatment for IBD.

The Clear Liquid Diet

The clear liquid diet is helpful during intense disease activity, in transition between intravenous feeding and solid food, following surgery, or in preparation for diagnostic tests. This diet is highly restrictive but provides some calories, prevents dehydration, and reduces intestinal activity.

Foods Allowed

- Fat free broth (made from poultry, fish, meat and/or vegetables)

- Bouillon
- Decaffeinated coffee
- Tea, herb teas
- Clear fruit juices and drinks (should be diluted to prevent diarrhea)
- Kool-aid (can be used to flavor commercial formulas)
- Popsicles (more nutritious when made from fruit juice or drinks)
- Gelatin (commercial products or homemade with clear juices)
- Carbonated beverages (without caffeine and allowed to flatten slightly)
- Honey, sugar, salt, flavorings

In addition, there are commercial semi-synthetic liquid diets which may be allowed on your clear liquid diet. The palatability of these products is generally poor, but creative use of flavorings can significantly improve their acceptability. A word of caution: if you use these formulas on your clear liquid diet, be sure to drink them slowly, since they are concentrated and may cause cramping or diarrhea. Always check with your doctor before using these formulas:

Citrotein	Precision HR
Vivonex Standard	Precision LR
Vivonex HN (high nitrogen)	Precision Isotonic
Vivonex TEN (Total Enteral Nutrition)	Criticare HN
	Vital HN

The Full Liquid Diet

The full liquid diet is traditionally used as a transition from clear liquids to solid food. This diet is more nutritious and palatable, and includes a greater variety of foods.

Foods Allowed:

Those on the Clear Liquid Diet *PLUS*:

- Milk, milk drinks, milk substitutes
- Cream and cream substitutes
- Eggs and egg substitutes used in custards, eggnogs, puddings, ice cream
- Fruit nectars
- Refined cooked cereals and strained whole grain cereals
- Puddings, ice cream, sherbet
- Vegetable juices
- Strained cream and vegetable soups

The full liquid diet can be implemented entirely using commercially prepared formulas instead of the foods listed, or they can be used as supplements to increase considerably the nutritional content of the diet.

A partial list of these products which can be taken orally includes:

Lactose Containing	*Lactose Free*
Meritene	Ensure, Ensure Plus, Ensure HN
Nutrament	Isotene HN
Carnation Instant Breakfast	Sustacal liquid, Sustacal HC (High calorie)
Sustacal powder	
Sustacal pudding	
Forta pudding	

Other products such as Isocal, Isocal HCN, Magnacal, Travasorb MCT, Osmolite and Travesorb Liquid are rather bland but are quite acceptable when mixed with flavorings, ice cream, etc.

The Lactose-Free Diet

Some individuals experience cramping, bloating and diarrhea when they consume milk because they are unable to adequately digest milk sugar (lactose). The full liquid diet is based on milk and milk products, so this poses a problem, but not an impossible one.

The intolerance to milk is caused by a lack of an intestinal enzyme called lactase, whose purpose is to break down lactose into simpler sugars that can be absorbed by the body. Those with diffuse small bowel disease may temporarily lack the enzyme, but in most it is an inherited trait that causes loss of the enzyme with age. While some people cannot consume even small amounts of milk, in most it is a dose-related phenomenon. Milk on cereal or ice cream may be fine, yet a whole glass of milk may produce symptoms. Yogurt is usually well-tolerated while buttermilk and acidophilus milk are not, even though they are cultured products as well.

Symptoms can often be prevented when the enzyme lactase is taken simultaneously with meals which contain lactose, or when commercially available lactase is added to milk.

Lactose-Free Foods:

Meat and Meat Substitute Group

- Eggs
- *Plain* meats of all kinds
- Poultry of all kinds
- Fish of all kinds (fresh or canned)
- Kosher hot dogs
- Cold cuts

Fruit and vegetable group:

- All plain fruits and vegetables (fresh, frozen or canned).

Bread and Cereal Group

- Bread and cereals made without milk or milk products
- Italian or French breads
- Pasta (macaroni, spaghetti, noodles)
- Crackers
- (Read labels carefully.)

Dairy Group

- Margarines which do not contain milk or milk products
- Non-dairy creamers
- Soy milk and other soy products

(Soy milk is becoming available commercially and *tofu* can be used as a meat substitute or in place of cream cheese or sour cream in many recipes. There is even a delectable milk-free ice cream substitute made from tofu, "Tofutti!")

Fats

- Salad dressings made without milk or milk products
- Vegetable oils
- Shortening
- Nut butters
- Nuts

Dairy Products with Minimal Lactose Content:

Lact-Aid treated milk: Lact-Aid, a commercially available lactase enzyme predigests the lactose in milk before use. The milk tastes slightly sweeter because lactose is broken into two simpler, sweeter-tasting sugars during digestion.

Milk can be treated at home using Lact-Aid drops or purchased pretreated in your supermarket dairy case under the Lact-Aid trademark. The company also makes cottage cheese and ice cream.

Margarine and Butter: Contain *trace* amounts of lactose.

Cheese: Blue, Brick, Camembert, Cheddar, Colby, Edam, Provolone, Swiss, pasteurized process American cheese all have "non-detectable" amounts of lactose. Cream cheese, cottage cheese and mozzarella contain small amounts of lactose but should not produce symptoms.

Ice Cream: The very "richest" kinds have the least lactose, since they contain more cream than milk.

The Bland Diet

The bland diet is defined as one which is "chemically and mechanically nonirritating." When given in small, frequent feedings, it may reduce symptoms caused by narrowing or active inflammation in the bowel. It is often unclear, however, which foods should be included or excluded because people differ in their food tolerances. As a result, the bland diet should be individualized. Be guided by the food list given by your physician or dietitian.

The bland diet generally *excludes:*

- Spices and highly seasoned foods: Black and red pepper, chili powder, mustard, nutmeg. (Cinnamon, allspice, cloves, paprika and herbs usually do not produce symptoms.)
- Caffeine in coffee, tea, colas and theobromine in chocolate.
- Alcohol
- Roughage: Especially raw fruits and vegetables with skins and small seeds, cereals and baked products made with unrefined flour, nuts, seeds, popcorn.

The Low Residue/Low Fiber Diet

People with disease located in the terminal ileum and/or colon may require what is called a low residue diet. A better name might be a "low roughage" diet, for the dietary goal is to provide a minimum of undigestable fiber which can block narrowed intestinal areas or irritate an inflamed colon. The problem is that the words *residue* and *fiber* are used interchangeably, yet are not really the same. Residue includes the total feces made up of undigested and unabsorbed food plus metabolic and bacterial products. For example, milk and prune juice contribute to fecal residue, yet contain no fiber. Fiber is that portion of plants that is not digested by the human intestinal tract. There are several kinds of fiber: cellulose, hemicellulose, lignin, pectins and algal polysaccharides, each with different properties. Foods that are high in cellulose, hemicellulose, and lignin may have difficulty passing through narrowed areas or may cause irritation. This kind of fiber is often called "roughage," hence the name "low roughage" diet. Remember, the foods which come from animals do not contain fiber (roughage).

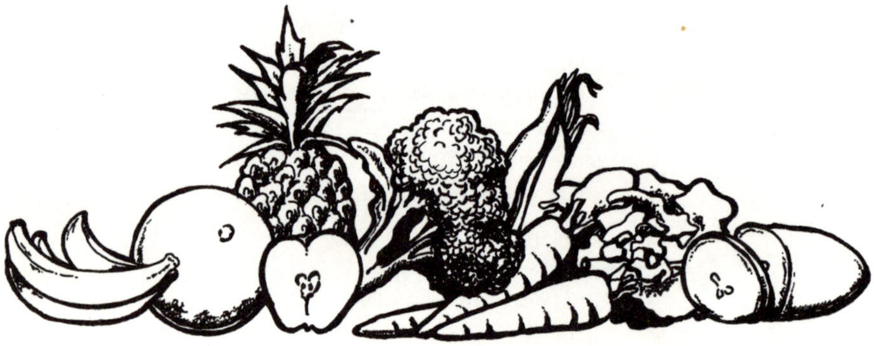

Minimal Roughage Diet	Restricted Roughage Diet
*Milk**: yogurt, cream	Same
Cheese: Cottage*, Cream*	Mild cheeses (e.g. cheddar, swiss)
Fats: Butter, margarine, vegetable oil, mayonnaise salad dressing	Same
Meat, poultry, fish: lean, tender beef, veal and lamb, chicken, turkey, fish (baked, boiled, broiled)	Same
Soups: Broths, noodle and rice soups, creamed soups	Same plus vegetable soups from those allowed
Vegetables: Potatoes (boiled, mashed, baked, unseasoned vegetable juices in limited amounts)	Potatoes plus cooked asparagus, green peas, green beans, spinach, squash, carrots
Fruits: Clear fruit juices in limited amounts (grape, cranberry, apple, orange*, lemonade*)	Fruit juices, cooked or canned fruits without skins or seeds, ripe bananas

Starches: Refined, enriched breads and cereals, macaroni, rice, noodles, spaghetti, crackers	Same
Desserts: Ices, ice cream*, pudding, custard*, gelatin, plain cake, candy and cookies without fruit or nuts	Same
Beverages: Tea, coffee*, carbonated beverages	Same
*Condiments**: Salt and sugar, mild spices	Same

(*if tolerated)

The Low Fat Diet

When Crohn's disease damages the ileum extensively, reabsorption of bile salts is greatly reduced. One important consequence of this is poor absorption of fats, fat soluble vitamins, calcium, and magnesium in the small intestine. A low fat diet is often prescribed to help alleviate the symptoms caused by this situation.

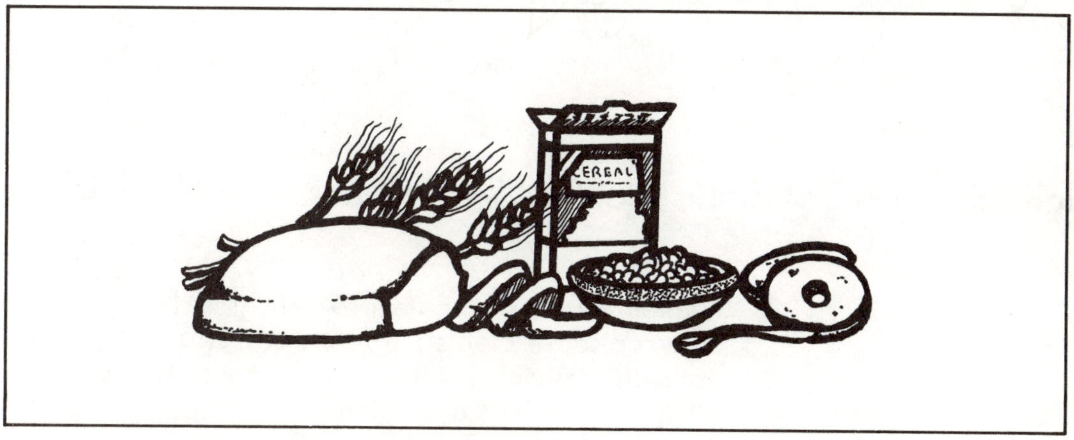

Food Allowed:

Meats, Fish, Poultry,
- Lean beef
- Lamb
- Veal
- Pork
- Organ meats
- Canadian bacon
- Poultry (without skin)
- Fish and shellfish (baked, boiled, broiled)

Eggs
- Whole eggs (3 weekly, including those used in cooking)
- Egg white as desired

Dairy
- Skim milk
- Buttermilk
- Low fat yogurt
- Low fat cheeses
- Low fat (1%) cottage cheese
- Mozzarella
- Special diet cheeses (Borden's Lite Line, Kraft Light & Lively)

Soups
- Fat free broth
- Bouillon
- Cream soups made with skim milk and allowed meats and vegetables

Starches
- Breads
- Pasta
- Cereals of all kinds
  - (Avoid waffles, doughnuts, coffee cakes)

Desserts
- Sherbet
- Fruit ice
- Gelatin
- Pudding made with skim milk
- Angel food cake
- Meringues
- Clear soft and hard candies
- Jelly
- Jam
- Syrup
- Marshmallows
  - (Not allowed:
  - Chocolate
  - Nuts
  - Ice Cream
  - Cake
  - Pie
  - Most cookies)

Fruits and Juices
- All kinds

Vegetables
- All except avocados

Fats
- 1-2 servings each meal
- Example of 1 serving:
  - 1 tsp. margarine, butter, oil, mayonnaise
  - 2 tbsp. half and half
  - 2 tsp. peanut butter
  - 1 strip crisp bacon

Beverages
- Coffee
- Tea
- Herb teas
- Carbonated beverages
- Cocoa made with skim milk
- Caffeine-free beverages
- Fruit juices
- Water

High Protein/High Calorie Diet

A high protein, high calorie diet is frequently recommended to correct weight loss, to stimulate growth in growth-impaired children and adolescents, to replenish protein stores caused by intestinal loss, and to prevent deficiencies during treatment. Although an ideal goal, this diet is sometimes difficult to follow because of other dietary restrictions, such as fat or roughage. Choosing "nutrient dense" foods—ones with the greatest nutrient/calorie ratios—can help fulfill calorie and nutrient goals. Happily, most Americans eat a very high protein diet, but unless calorie levels are adequate, the protein is used for energy rather than for the building of body tissue.

Diet Outline:
The daily diet plan should include the following foods or their nutritive equivalents in age-appropriate amounts:

- *Milk*: (Whole) 4 servings (1 serving = 1 cup)
- *Meat*: (Or meat substitutes) 2 large servings (1 serving = 3-4 ounces)
- *Vegetables*: (4 servings—including one green or yellow, one potato or substitute, and two others (1 serving = ½ cup)
- *Fruits*: 3 servings—including one citrus (1 serving = ½ cup)
- *Enriched grains*: 6 servings—including cereal, breads, pasta (1 serving = ½ cup of pasta or 1 slice bread)
- *Fortified margarine or butter*: 5 servings
- *Desserts and sweets*: As desired

Supplemental formulas (listed on the full liquid diet) can be used with meals and snacks or in preparing soups, casseroles, desserts, milk shakes. Extra powdered milk can be added to creamed dishes, gravies, milk, cottage cheese, dips, peanut butter. There are protein supplements with little lactose content which can be used similarly (Casec, Propac, Pro-mix). Glucose and glucose polymers (e.g. Polycose, Controlyte) are less sweet than table sugar (sucrose) and can be used in larger amounts without making foods too sweet.

MCT oil contains almost 8 calories per cc., and can be added in tiny amounts to many foods (soups, casseroles, sauces, desserts, milkshakes, juice), significantly increasing their caloric content. This oil is almost tasteless and less "oily" than other fats, but it does have two drawbacks. It can produce diarrhea when used in large amounts, and it is more expensive.

The high protein/high calorie diet is best implemented using small, frequent meals rather than large ones. Snacks become "meals" in their importance.

Protein Food Equivalents:
(Each serving provides approximately 7 grams of protein. Fat and calorie values will vary.)

Meats, poultry, fish
(1 ounce portion)
- Canned fish—1/4 cup
- Sardines—3
- Clams, oysters, shrimp, scallops—5
- Cold cuts—1 slice (1/8 inch thick)
- Hot dog—1

Dairy products
- Milk—1 cup
- Yogurt—1 cup
- Cheese—1 ounce (1 slice of most cheeses)
  - Grated parmesan—3 tbsp.
  - Cottage cheese—1/4 cup
- Pudding, ice cream or sherbet
  1 (generous) cup

Eggs
- One

Nuts and Seeds
- Almonds—25
- Brazil nuts—10
- Cashews—12-16
- Peanuts or peanut butter
  2 tbsp.
- Seeds—3 tbsp.

Legumes and lentils
- 1/2 cup cooked
- Tofu—1/3 cup

Grains
- Bread—4 slices
- Cereal—1 1/2 cups
- Rice, potatoes, pasta—1 1/2 cups cooked
- Pop tarts—4

Miscellaneous
- Pizza—1/8-10 inch pizza
- Tacos—1/2
- Macaroni and cheese 1/2—1 cup
- Pot pie—1/2

*Vegetarians should check with their physician and/or nutritionist to assure the adequacy of their diets and correct complimentary proteins.

II. Food Sources of Important Vitamins

Vitamin A:

Animal sources contain pre-formed vitamin A:

Liver	Cheese
Eggs	Butter and Cream
Milk	Fish liver oils

Plant sources contain carotenes which are converted to vitamin A in the body:

Dark green leafy vegetables

Broccoli	Asparagus
Spinach	Green peas

Yellow vegetables and fruits

Carrots	Sweet potatoes
Peaches	Winter squash
Oranges	Cantaloupe
	Tomatoes

Vitamin D:

- SUNLIGHT!!!!!!!!
- Liver
- Fish liver oils
- Fortified milk
- Butter and fortified margarines
- Eggs
- Fortified cereals (check labels)

Vitamin C (Ascorbic Acid):

Fruits	*Vegetables*
Citrus fruits	Broccoli
Strawberries	Tomatoes (raw), tomato juice
Melon	Dark green leafy vegetables
Bananas	Cabbage
Apples	Potatoes
	Green peppers
	Asparagus

Folic Acid (Folacin):

A special kind of anemia results from a deficiency of folic acid. This may occur when sulfasalazine interferes with its absorption. Supplemental amounts are frequently given along with this medication. There are excellent food sources as well, but care must be taken in cooking and storage, since folic acid is easily destroyed by heat, light and air. The name folic acid or folacin is derived from the word "foliage," since green leafy vegetables are among its most important sources. Those on a restricted roughage diet cannot eat "foliage," and may be better off using a supplement.

Food Rich in Folic Acid (Folacin):

- Liver
- Beets
- Corn
- Frozen peas
- Legumes and Lentils
- Parsnips
- Frozen orange juice
- Green leafy vegetables:
  - Broccoli
  - Brussel sprouts
  - Endive
  - Spinach
  - Romaine

Vitamin B-12:
Vitamin B-12 deficiency in IBD is commonly caused by ileal disease or resection of the ileum, the site of absorption of this vitamin. It can also be the result of a vegetarian diet, since meat, fish and poultry are the principal dietary sources of this vitamin. Your physician will obtain serum levels periodically if you are in danger of becoming deficient and/or perform a Schilling Test to assess your ability to absorb vitamin B-12. True deficiency of this vitamin is usually treated by monthly injections of the vitamin rather than with diet or oral supplements.

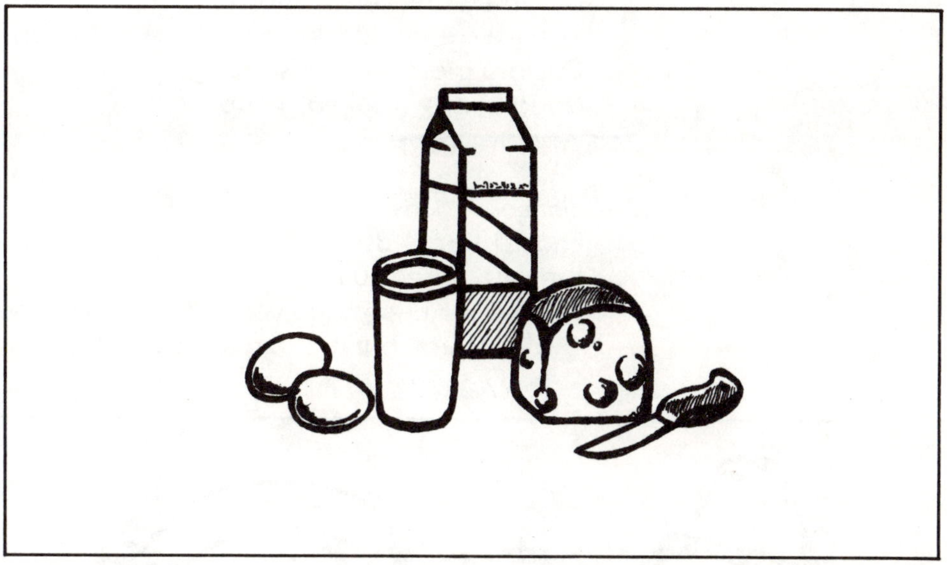

III. Food Sources of Important Minerals

Calcium:
An adequate intake of calcium is important for everyone. For the person with IBD, it is even more essential, because IBD can cause increased losses and dietary restrictions may decrease the availability of this nutrient. Without milk in some form, it is difficult to get enough calcium, and supplements may be necessary. Check with your physician or nutritionist to find your requirement for calcium. Use the following table to combine foods that will provide that amount or ask to have a suitable supplement prescribed that will allow you to meet your need for calcium.

Foods Rich in Calcium:
The following foods contain 300 milligrams of calcium:

- Milk: All kinds (skim, whole, buttermilk)—1 cup
  - Dry Skim Milk Powder—1/3 cup
- Yogurt: 1 cup
- Sardines: 3 ounces

The following foods contain 200 milligrams of calcium:

Cheese: American, cheddar, brick, processed cheese food—1 ounce

Ice cream or ice milk: (Regular kinds)—1 cup
(Richer ice creams—e.g. Baskin-Robbins—contain only 100 mg per cup.)

Cheese souffle: 1 serving (3¼″ x 3¼″ x 2″)

Cooked greens: 1 cup

The following foods contain 150 milligrams of calcium:

Pudding: All kinds (made from mixes, rice, bread)—½ cup

Baked custard: ½ cup

Pizza: 1 serving (¼ of 10″ diameter cheese pizza, ¼″ thick)

Cream soup made with milk: Tomato, chicken, asparagus, etc.)—1 cup

The following foods contain 100 milligrams of calcium:

Cheese: All kinds—1 cubic inch

Cottage cheese: ½ cup

Creamed Chicken: 1 cup

Rich ice cream: (Baskin-Robbins type) 1 cup

Custard pie: (⅙ pie) 1 serving

Dried beans: (cooked) 1 cup

~~Peanuts: 1 cup~~

Miscellaneous Foods

Eggs: 1 large—30 mg

Bread: 1 slice—20 mg

Nuts, dried beans and vegetable greens contain large amounts of calcium, but it is in a form which is not readily used by the body.

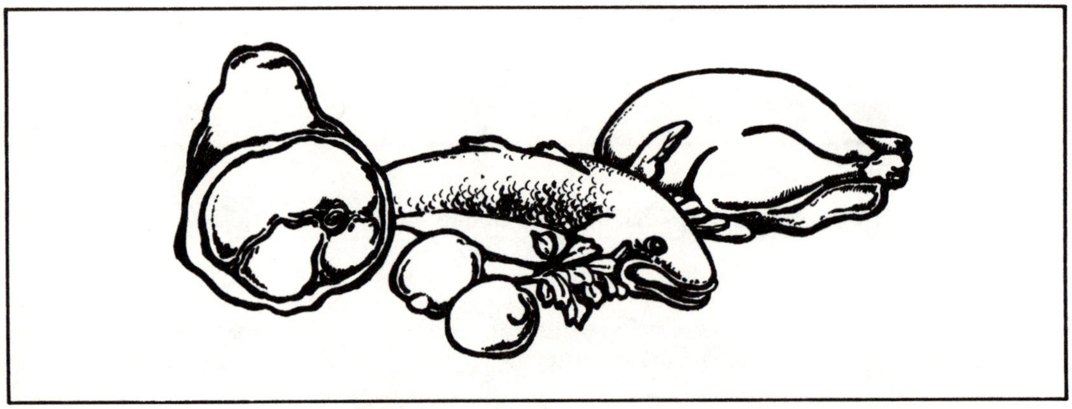

Iron:

Many people with IBD are frequently anemic. There are a number of possible causes for this, and anemia cannot usually be treated with diet alone. Iron supplements are necessary, but can cause bowel irritation and cramping. It is therefore helpful to have some information about ways to increase the amount of iron in the food we eat. There are two kinds of iron in food—heme and non-heme iron. Heme iron is found in red meat. Non-heme iron is found mostly in plant foods, and is less available to the body. Eating non-heme iron foods with meat, fish or poultry will increase its absorption. Eating a food rich in vitamin C will also increase the absorption of both heme and non-heme iron. This information will allow you to plan meals which will enhance the absorption and availability of the iron in all your foods.

Iron Equivalents:

(Each serving of the foods listed below yields approximately 1 milligram of iron.)

- Liver: 1/2 ounce
- Beef: 1 ounce
- Egg: 1
- Chicken: 3 ounces
- Legumes and lentils: 1/3 cup cooked
- Greens: 1/3 cup (including spinach)
- Potatoes: 1 medium
- Rice, spaghetti, noodles: 1 cup
- Prunes: 4
- Raisins: 1/6 cup
- Pork, lamb: 1 ounce
- Hot dogs: 1 (8 per pound)
- Oysters: 1 medium
- Fish: (Fresh, canned tuna, sardines, salmon)–3 oz.
- Fishsticks: 10
- Most fruits: 1 cup
- Most breads: 2 slices
- Many prepared cereals: 1 oz. (Check labels)
- Milk: 10 cups

Zinc:

It has been suggested that zinc deficiency may have a role in IBD, and that zinc supplementation might be considered in its treatment, especially in children with growth impairment. While the role of zinc in IBD is still unclear, it is important as a component of many enzymes in the body and it plays an essential role in DNA and RNA synthesis.

Zinc deficiency can be produced by malabsorption. Foods high in fiber can also interfere with its absorption. In additon, zinc, iron and copper can compete with each other for incorporation into compounds in the body. For this reason the *ratio* of these metals to each other is very sensitive, and supplementation should be undertaken *only* with the advice of your physician and/or nutritionist.

Food Rich in Zinc:

Animal Foods

- Beef, lamb, pork, veal
- Chicken, turkey (dark meat)
- Liver, heart
- Crab, lobster, oysters, shrimp
- Cheese (cheddar, American, gouda, mozzarella, munster, Swiss)

Plant Foods

- Legumes and lentils
- Bran
- Nuts
- Green peas
- Grains (wheat, rice, wheat germ and products made from these)

Summary

Deficiencies of essential nutrients may occur in IBD depending on the location and extent of disease. The primary nutrients are: protein, calories, vitamins A, D, C, B-12 and folic acid; calcium, iron and zinc. No doubt, other deficiencies occur. The best protection is to eat a variety of foods from the basic four food groups, choosing sources that are rich in the nutrients you need and conform to the dietary modifications you require.

Sometimes vitamin and/or mineral supplements are needed for optimal health. Be guided by the advice of your physician or nutritionist in your choice of supplements.

11

Sports And The Person With IBD

Sports and physical exercise are important both in the maintenance and restoration of health. People with IBD are like all people in their need for physical exercise, yet are different because of the special precautions they must take as a result of the disease or the effects of medical and surgical treatments.

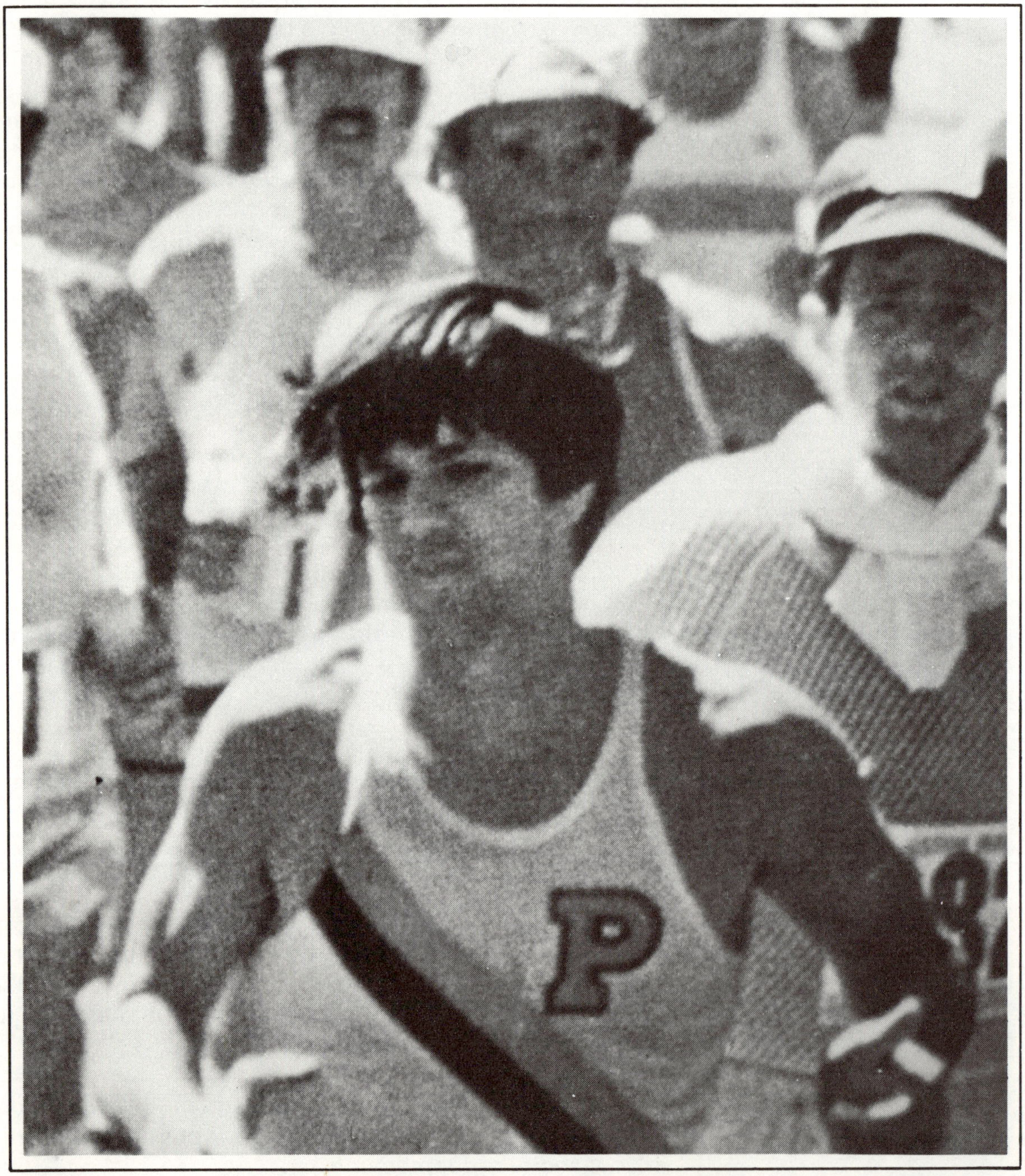

The Benefits of Exercise

Until about 15 years ago, most people were spectators at sporting events. Very few actually participated in vigorous physical exercise. Most people seemed to confine their physical activity to a social game of golf or tennis. It was only with popularization of the concept of "aerobics" that large numbers of people throughout the world began to jog, run, walk, cycle and swim.

Aerobic activity is defined as activity in which the work of the heart is raised to a sub-maximal level of activity and oxygen demands during this activity are supplied by the intake of oxygen by the lungs. The pace is such that it is still possible to talk during this activity. Numerous studies have demonstrated that people who take the time to engage in aerobic exercise will derive a sense of well-being and accomplishment. A study of Harvard alumni showed that college athletes who did not maintain their state of fitness were at higher risk from coronary artery disease than college non-athletes who later entered an aerobic program and became fit. Other studies have demonstrated that sedentary individuals have a higher mortality rate from coronary artery disease than active individuals. Although no studies have shown that people who exercise live longer, all studies report an increased sense of well-being among those who do exercise.

The person with IBD may benefit from exercise even more than the healthy individual. Physical activity such as walking, jogging, swimming, cycling, and rowing tends to reverse some of the debilitating aspects of the disease, such as muscle weakness. Exercise also counteracts muscle wasting and calcium loss from bone caused by prolonged bed rest both in and out of the hospital. An additional benefit of vigorous exercise for the person with IBD is the sense of exhilaration or "runner's high," which tends to lift the spirits in depressed individuals. Some researchers suggest that prolonged exercise triggers the release of opiate-like hormones from the brain (called endorphins or encephalins), which may be responsible for the improved mood changes.

Psychologically, exercise can help people with IBD erase negative feelings about themselves and help them learn to trust their bodies again.

Nutrition and Exercise

All individuals require an adequate supply of calories as well as appropriate amounts of carbohydrates, fats, proteins, fluids, vitamins, calcium, potassium and trace elements (see Chapters 9 and 10). During prolonged physical activity, energy is derived first from glycogen, (carbohydrates that are stored in muscle). Later, energy is derived from the breakdown of fats. If these sources are unavailable, the body then breaks down protein to supply energy needs.

For this reason, carbohydrates should be the main component of the diet and should primarily be complex starches which take longer to break down, rather than sugars. Fats are essential for both IBD and non-IBD individuals and should be of the polyunsaturated or monounsaturated variety. If fat malabsorption is a problem, medium chain triglycerides (MCT oil) can be substituted. Proteins are essential for growth and maintenance of body tissues. The body's need for protein rises with increased physical activity, fever, chronic disease activity, and infection, as well as with increased protein losses in diarrhea.

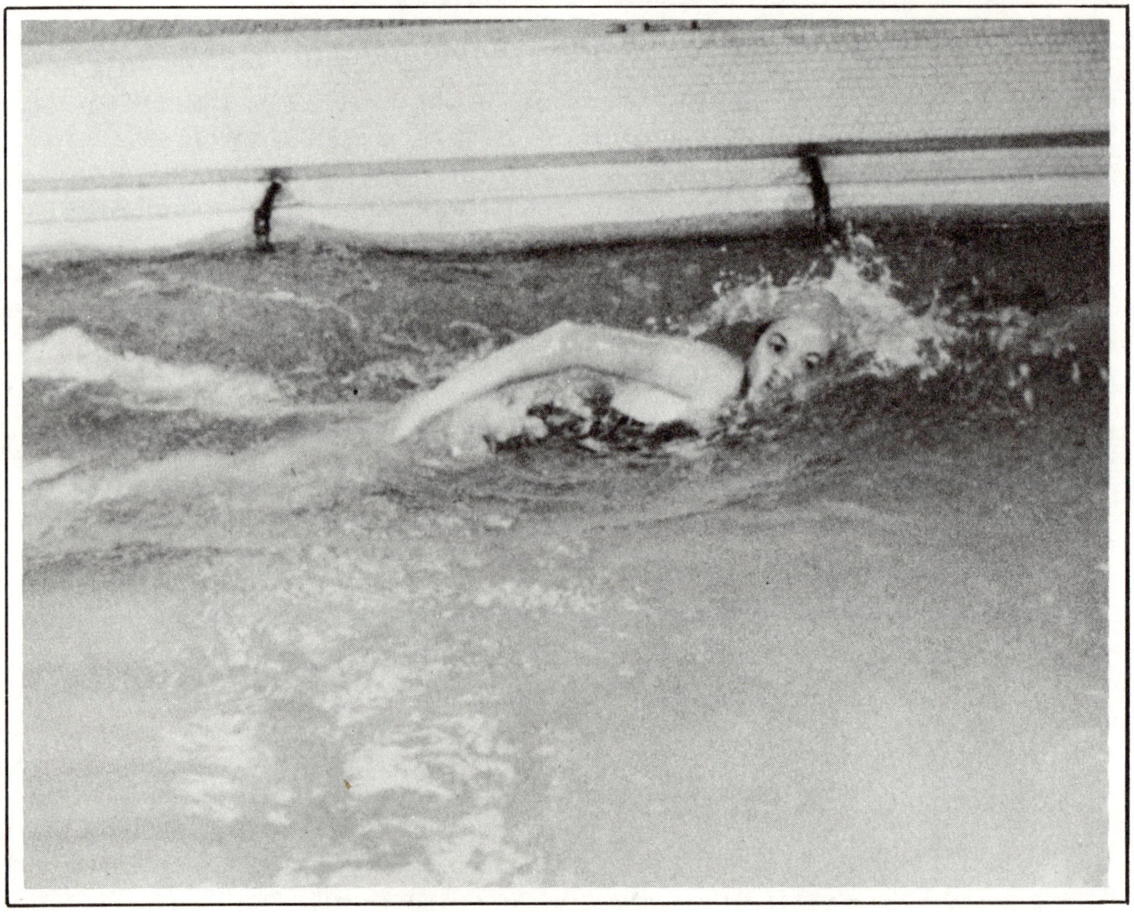

Considerable amounts of body fluids are lost with exercise, especially in the person having diarrhea and the person with an ileostomy. The exerciser who has IBD should know that it is often not enough to rely on thirst alone to replace lost fluids.

Although most healthy individuals require no dietary supplements, there are times when specific vitamins and minerals are lost and should be replaced. (This subject is covered extensively in Chapter 10.) People with IBD who take steroids tend to become potassium-deficient, may experience muscle cramping and weakness, and may be unable to tolerate vigorous exercise. Oral potassium supplements (or foods high in potassium) can be taken on the advice of the doctor. Likewise, those who avoid milk products because of lactase deficiency may need to take calcium supplements.

The help of a dietician or nutritionist can be extremely valuable for the person with IBD. This is especially true if you are about to begin a program of vigorous exercise.

What Sport Should I Choose?

Non-spectator sports can be grouped into four categories: non-aerobic sports (like golf or tennis), weight training, contact sports, and endurance (aerobic) sports. Golf and tennis provide healthy outdoor exercise, social interaction and a sense of accomplishment for the person with IBD. Weight training, using free weights or machines such as the Nautilus or Universal, can help in rebuilding certain muscle groups which have become weakened by disease or by the use of corticosteroids. In this chapter, Peter Nielsen, Mr. International Universe, describes how he used weight training to overcome muscle weakness caused by the Crohn's disease he has had since childhood.

Contact sports, like football or wrestling, may expose the person with IBD to injury, especially if bones are weakened by steroid therapy, or if there has been ostomy surgery. Nevertheless, Rolf Benirschke and Uwe von Schamann, both ulcerative colitis sufferers, continue to play active professional football using proper precautions. Later in the chapter, Benirschke explains how a graduated program of exercise helped him gain back strength following his 1979 surgery.

Endurance (aerobic) sports such as jogging, cycling, swimming, or rowing cause no physical contact and therefore little chance for injury. These sports strengthen muscles which have become weak from disuse, improve cardiovascular performance, and help the person with IBD to achieve a sense of well-being. They also increase the deposition of calcium into previously weakened bone. During periods of inclement weather, indoor tracks or stationary bicycles can be utilized to sustain the exercise program.

Together with your physician, you should select from the sports and activities mentioned above those which will be most helpful, physically and psychologically, in the maintenance of health.

Special Precautions for the Person with IBD

Anemia is common in many people with active IBD. The anemia may be caused by inadequate amounts of iron in the diet or by exessive intestinal losses of iron, vitamin B-12 or folic acid. Obviously, attempts should be made to correct the anemia with the appropriate supplement. Many runners, even those without IBD, may become somewhat anemic. Whatever causes the anemia diminishes the body's ability to supply oxygen to muscle and other tissues, causing you to tire easily or to become breathless. You should work with your physician to rectify the anemia and slow the pace of your activity until the problem is resolved.

Many persons who exercise develop an increased need to move their bowels and some even develop diarrhea. This may be due to the release into the bloodstream of certain hormones which increase intestinal motility. People with IBD should be warned that this may occur during exercise and should not fear such an occurrence. Some people prevent this problem by moving their bowels prior to activity. Those with severe diarrhea from IBD may find that a Lomotil or Imodium tablet taken prior to exercising provides sufficient protection.

Dehydration during vigorous exercise is a special danger to the person with IBD who may already be losing fluid and electrolytes with active diarrhea. Danger signs to watch for are fatigue, dizziness, decreased urine output, and muscle cramps. If any of these signs occur during exercise, it is best to contact your physician immediately.

The use of corticosteroids causes special problems for anyone engaging in vigorous exercise. Weight gain from fluid retention causes a greater strain on the body. Muscles become weaker, bones become softer, and skin becomes thinner and more easily bruised. Calcium and potassium losses may accelerate electrolyte imbalance and other metabolic problems.

Before beginning any exercise program, the person with IBD should consult his or her physician. The physician is responsible for coordinating the medical treatment program and will be aware of any reasons why such an exercise program should *not* be started. It may also be advisable to consult experts in exercise training or sports medicine. Many centers now have training programs for "beginning exercisers," or for those with medical problems.

Advice from the Athletes...

Rolf Benirschke, Placekicker for the San Diego Chargers

On taking steroids...

"When I was sick and my body was fighting the disease, it was very difficult for me to keep my weight on. Everything I ate went into fighting the inflammation, and very little of it to laying down any muscle protein. This was further retarded by taking prednisone, a catabolic steroid, which breaks down muscle fibers. I'm not sure how you counteract that. I think that this is one of the really tough things that athletes with IBD have to deal with. While the prednisone is necessary to keep the inflammation under control, it is also very difficult if you are trying to maintain an athletic regimen."

On building up strength after surgery...

"You start by doing little things, like walking. In the hospital, I started with walking to the nurse's station and back three times a day. By the time I was released from the hospital, my goal was to get up in the morning and walk to my neighbor's house and back. Each day I added another house. Next, I started some weight training. I think if you just listen to your body, and don't overdo it initially, your body will tell you how quickly to progress.

"I wouldn't recommend any one particular program of exercise. The only way you can definitely build up your strength by exercising is to find something that you enjoy, whether it is riding a bicycle or playing tennis, and to try to keep at it."

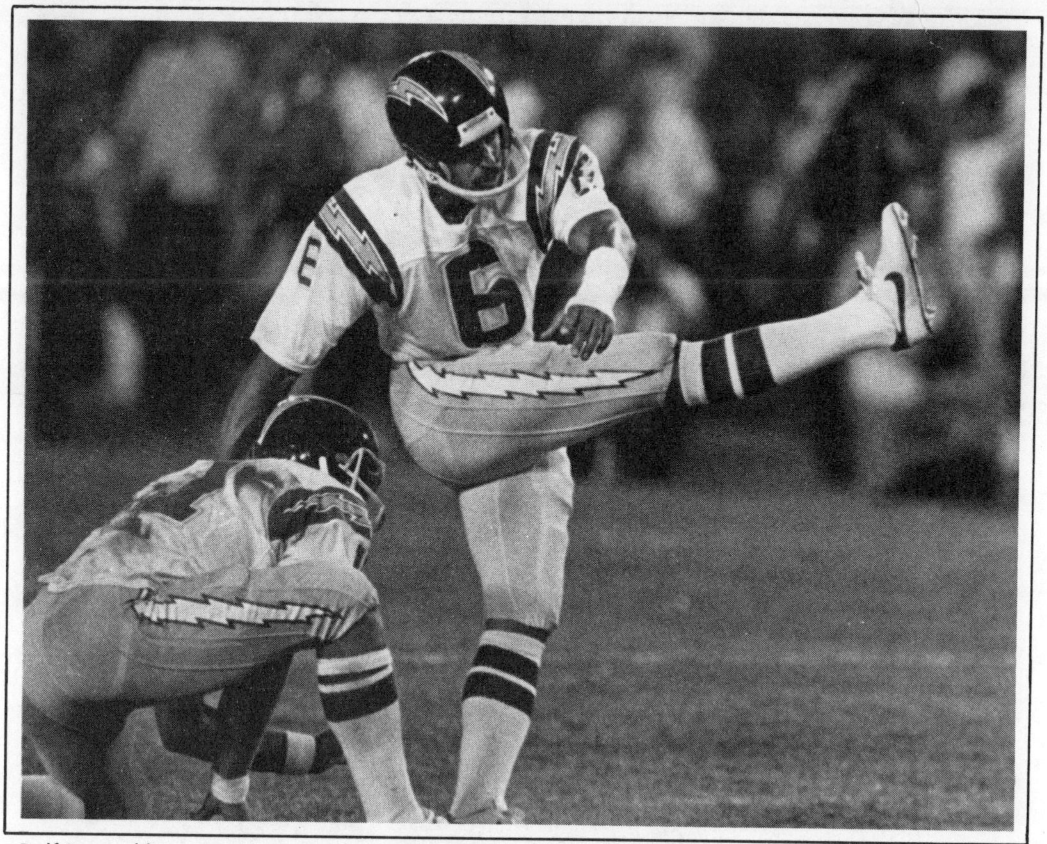

Rolf Benirschke in action on the football field—Photo by Sam Stone, San Diego Chargers

On the fear of surgery...

"I have a career that demands physical excellence. I didn't have surgery earlier because I was afraid that it would end my career. So I tried to put it off as long as possible. What I have learned is that I really jeopardized my life. I really waited too long and got so sick that the surgery became an emergency, and there were complications. As a result, I almost died. If I had listened to my body a little earlier, I might not have risked my life the way I did.

"After surgery, I was really scared. I didn't know what else to do. If I was not going to get back and live the kind of life I had been living, I didn't want to live. That kind of life meant being athletic...I read a lot of motivational books about people who had been down and out–not necessarily from IBD–and how they dealt with it. As a result, I have to say that I developed a faith that I didn't originally have and that helped me a lot."

Editors' Note

In 1982, Rolf Benirschke underwent his third IBD-related operation which resulted in the removal of his entire colon and rectum, and the construction of a permanent continent ileostomy (Kock pouch). Since the surgery is considered the "cure" for ulcerative colitis, he is now considered to be free of the disease.

Despite any setbacks due to his illness, Benirschke's football career has been consistently successful. In 1983, he was named NFL Man of the Year. In 1984, he was cited as the second most accurate kicker in the League. As Chairman of the NFIC Sports Council, Benirschke has enlisted the support of over one hundred fellow athletes in the fight against Crohn's disease and ulcerative colitis.

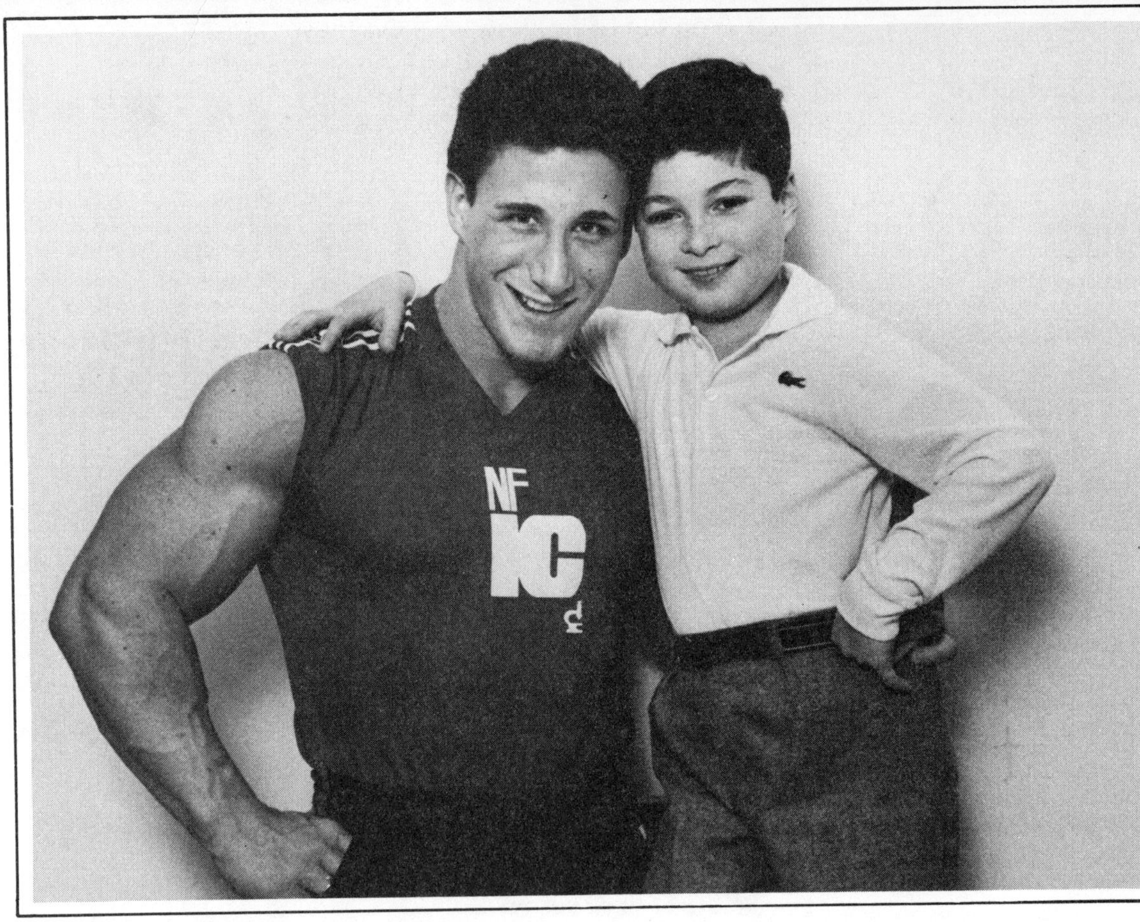

Peter Nielsen and friend—Photo by Stanley Seligson

Peter Nielsen, Mr. International Universe

On exercise...
"An exercise program for people with inflammatory bowel disease can work in so many ways. The mind is the most vital muscle in the body. You have to take the negative energy and turn it into positive energy, and learn to stop feeling sorry for yourself. Walk, play basketball, anything you really *want* or *can* do."

On getting started in bodybuilding...
"I got into bodybuilding because I had lost so much weight–from 145 pounds down to 86 pounds–from the Crohn's disease. I was so fragile that the doctor recommended something to build me up. What I really wanted to do was to prove to everyone that I could use my handicap as an advantage instead of a disadvantage. I wanted to be recognized as Number One, so I picked a sport where I could *be* Number One.

"Having Crohn's disease is the main reason why I'm successful at what I do. Because I lost so much weight and became so frightened at such a young age, something inside me made me want to prove myself to everyone who said I'd never gain weight or be normal again."

On competing...
"Before a competition, I go into my own little world. I start thinking about how I felt when I was sick. I'm on stage because I want everyone to know that I started with a handicap and overcame it. I have the edge. That edge, that desire to win, is a positive result of my illness.

"When I'm competing, I follow these rules:

1. I try not to eat much before traveling.
2. I'm extra careful of what I eat *while* I'm traveling.
3. I don't eat anything before I compete.
4. I travel prepared. I bring extra medicine and foods I know I can eat in my hotel room. That makes me feel more secure."

On learning when to stop...

"As I get older and more mature, I am learning when to stop. I always go the limit until I can't go any more. I do listen to my body. I know how my body feels and when something feels wrong. When you have to stop, you stop—no excuses. My goal now is to keep my body and my head in good working order."

Editors' Note

At the age of 23, Peter Nielsen has accumulated more titles than anyone in the history of the sport of bodybuilding. As the newest member of NFIC's Sports Council, he visits public schools in the New York area, telling young people about his fight against Crohn's disease, and delivering his message of hope.

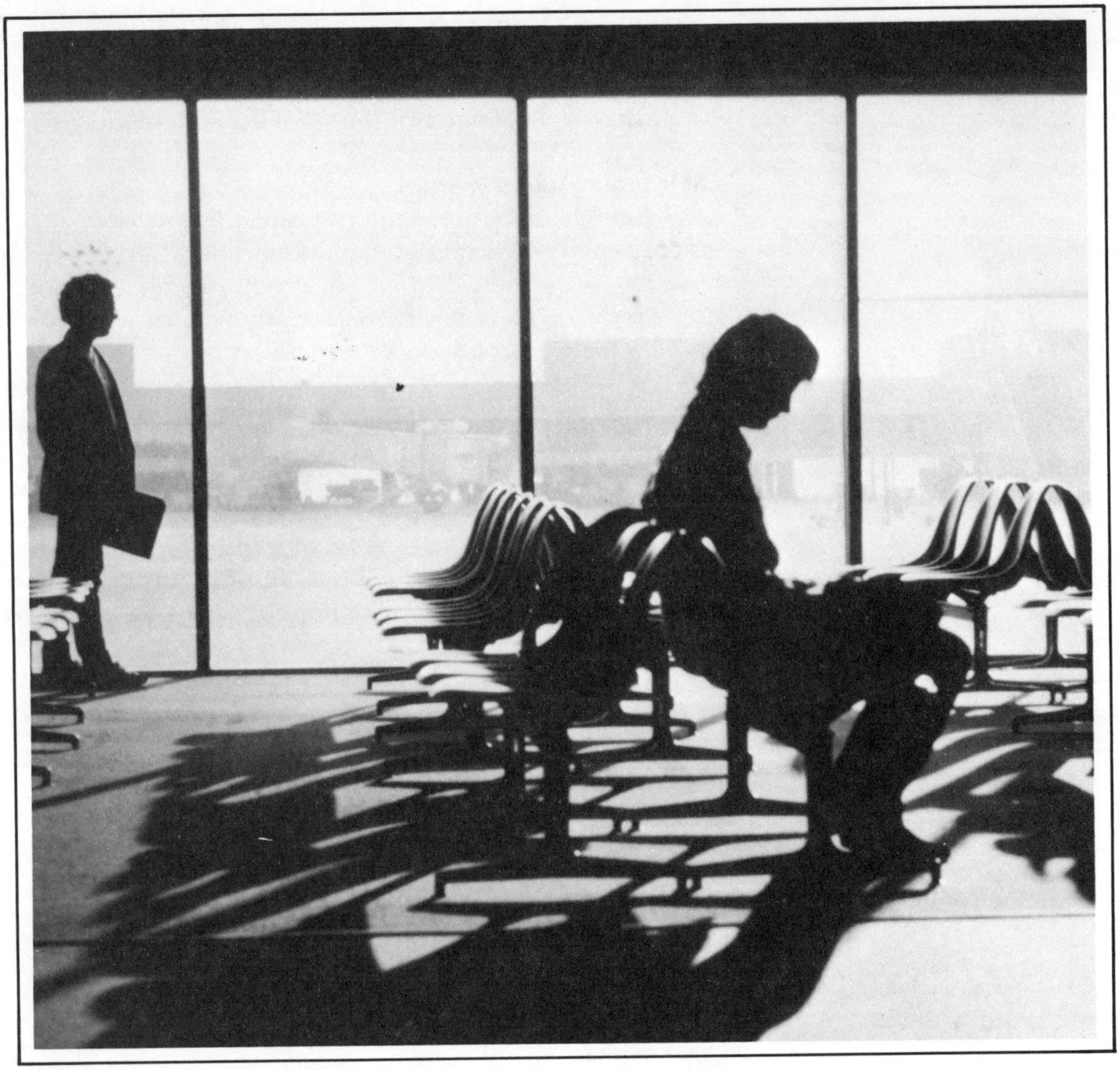

12 Traveling With IBD

All of us enjoy our freedom to travel within the United States and abroad, IBD sufferers no less than others. The IBD sufferer cannot leave illness at home along with the pets, so plans have to be made and answers prepared to the question "what if...?"

Traveling within the United States

The United States, with its enormous geographical and climatic contrast, offers wonderful opportunities for travel and exploration which many of us tend to overlook. For travelers who have IBD, there is the comfortable knowledge that the drinking water throughout the country is pure and that the risks of traveler's diarrhea and food poisoning are remote. There should also be no problem with regard to health insurance coverage and there is a national standard of treatment for the complications of IBD if a flare-up of symptoms should occur.

Before traveling within the U.S., however, it is a good idea to discuss your plans with your physician to be sure that you are fit enough to make your planned trip. You should take with you enough current medication to last the length of the trip. Take along your physician's telephone number in your wallet so that you can contact his/her office in any sort of emergency. Also be sure to carry your insurance card, just in case. Let your doctor know where in particular you plan to visit, as he/she can often give you the name of a colleague in that part of the country. Doctors who treat IBD usually know good reliable physicians in every part of the country who would be able to handle any type of IBD emergency. If your case is particularly complex, it would be wise for your doctor to give you a typed summary describing your history, physical findings and current medications.

These comments also apply to travel to Canada, Bermuda, Puerto Rico and the U.S. Virgin Islands. However, if you plan to travel to Canada or Bermuda, check with your insurance carrier just to be sure that medical expenses are covered if the need were to arise.

Travel by car and camper is easy and generally poses few problems. Likewise, bus and train travel are relatively comfortable. Remember to find out in advance if the tour bus has a toilet. Long air trips, such as coast-to-coast or to Hawaii, can be tiring. It is always a good plan to try to get an aisle seat, so make arrangements ahead of time with the airline. Airlines are very helpful with special diets, but they need a few days prior notification of your needs.

If you plan any really vigorous or new exercise such as skiing or hiking in the National Parks, discuss this with your doctor and be sure that you know your own limits. Any back-packing trip where medical care is unavailable should be seriously discussed before you make final plans.

Overseas Travel and Travel to Latin America

Foreign travel demands fairly careful planning not only for your trip, but also for the possibility of trouble with your IBD.

Travel to Western Europe, Scandinavia, most of Eastern Europe, Australia, New Zealand and South Africa carries little risk of exposure to unpleasant illness. Travel to Latin America, the Caribbean and less developed countries does have its risks, especially if you leave the standard "tourist circuit." Cruises rarely expose you to any illness worse than sunburn and weight gain! However, it is wise to inquire in advance about the medical facilities available on board the ship.

Travel to the tropics often requires special immunizations, so again check with your doctor long before you leave on a trip. Find out about the risk of malaria, which is unfortunately making a major comeback in Africa and Asia. Hepatitis can be a risk in the developing countries as well as in the Mediterranean, so injections against hepatitis A and B may be recommended. Next, contact your medical insurance carrier and find out if there are forms to complete to keep up your coverage when you are out of the U.S.

After you have carried out these preliminary steps, you must get down to your basic medical needs for the trip. Make sure you have all your medications in their appropriate vials, properly labelled. Customs officers can be very suspicious when faced with pills not contained in vials with your name on them, so keep all medicines in separate individual vials. Do not take samples and try not to use any type of pill box, except for use on the plane. Always carry your medications with you through customs. Do not check them in with your baggage! If you need narcotic medications, such as tincture of opium or codeine tablets, be doubly certain that the bottle or vial is labelled and that the label is secure. Let your pharmacist know that you will be taking your medicines out of the country.

How to Keep Healthy when Traveling

Diarrhea afflicts one out of three U.S. travelers to less developed countries. The odds are in your favor that you won't come down with "turista," "Delhi belly," or "Montezuma's revenge." However, there are guidelines which will cut down on the risk of contracting diarrhea, which is usually caused by an organism as such enterotoxigenic (entero = intestinal, toxi = toxin or poison, genic = producing) *Escherichia coli*. This organism is passed to travelers by fecal contamination of water or food. The guidelines are:

- Avoid tap water and all beverages containing water served in a pitcher. Water that has been boiled thoroughly (such as for tea) is acceptable, as are commercially bottled beverages. Be sure to open all bottles yourself or have them opened in your presence to be sure that tap water is not added.
- Avoid all ice and ice cream.
- Avoid raw vegetables and salads.
- Avoid uncooked dairy products such as milk and cheese unless you are sure that they are pasteurized and prepared under sterile conditions.

- Never eat food from vendors' carts.
- Never eat prepared foods such as potato salad and cocktail canapes–even in elegant surroundings.
- Peel all fruits yourself.
- Peel egg shells yourself.

Most resort and business hotels in lesser developed countries have special water purification equipment, but always check with hotel staff to find out about their facilities. When in doubt, stick to bottled mineral water, even when you brush your teeth. Bath water may not be purified, so don't swallow water when showering. Be careful when swimming in fresh water, in dubious swimming pools, or where the ocean may be polluted.

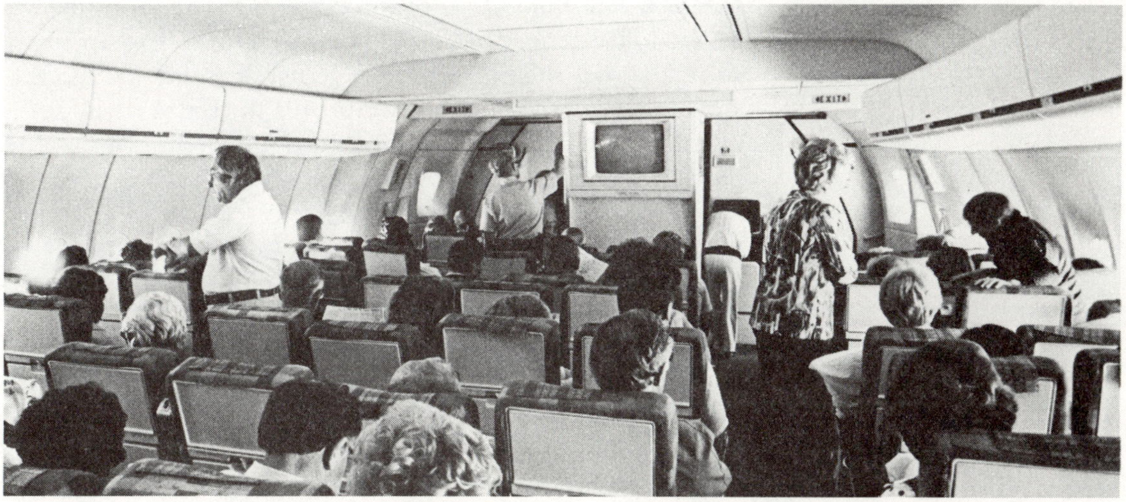

There are two schools of thought about taking medicine to prevent traveler's diarrhea. A recent National Institutes of Health consensus development panel recommended that in healthy individuals the risk of using preventive medication outweights the benefits, and that antimicrobial medicines are better used for *treatment* of traveler's diarrhea than for prevention. The other opinion would offer preventive medicines to those who would like to take them after careful consideration of possible side effects.

The IBD patient has to be given special consideration since a two to four day bout with diarrhea may be very unpleasant and demoralizing. Small doses of the antibiotic doxycycline have been effective in preventing diarrhea in U.S. citizens traveling abroad and the cheaper antimicrobial trimethoprim, with or without sulfamethoxazole, is also effective. (Patients taking sulfasalazine would be wise to *avoid* taking the trimethoprim and sulfonamide combination.) These drugs are also effective in treating diarrhea, as is Pepto Bismol in very large doses.

Gastroenterologists differ in their advice to IBD patients about taking any of the above medicines to protect against traveler's diarrhea, so each IBD sufferer should discuss this carefully with his/her doctor. There are occasional side effects to worry about, especially with doxycycline, which can cause rashes and increased sensitivity to the sun. Pediatric gastroenterologists may recommend a preventive dose of trimethoprim for their young patients when they travel into the less developed countries, but here again, side effects must be considered.

If you do come down with traveler's diarrhea when on a trip, remember to drink plenty of fluids and take extra salt to prevent dehydration. Water or weak tea is perhaps preferable to citrus drinks or soda (both of which may increase motility and could accentuate the diarrhea). Lukewarm fluids are preferable to ice cold beverages, which also may increase diarrhea. Such standard antidiarrheal medications as Lomotil and Imodium relieve cramps and reduce general discomfort. Be sure to follow your doctor's instructions regarding these medications and their dosages to avoid any possibility of complications of your IBD that could be caused by overusage of these preparations. Remember that the illness is often short-lived, with more than half of patients improving within two days and three-quarters within four days.

Travel out of the U.S. also exposes us to different, more exotic foods and cooking preparations. Cruise ships and international hotel chains provide "international" cuisine which is much like standard American fare, but local restaurants and cafés may serve food which is much spicier or much oilier than what we are used to. If spices or greasy foods do not sit well in your stomach or intestines at home, they probably won't when you are on vacation. In tropical countries, there is an abundance of fruit available, so be certain not to overindulge in roughage which can cause looseness of the stool or aggravate an underlying bowel obstruction.

Some IBD sufferers may worry that the risks of travel to Latin America and other less developed countries are going to make them so anxious that their trip will be spoiled. In that case, consider a cruise to the Pacific Coast of Mexico or in the Caribbean. Hawaii, the Virgin Islands and Puerto Rico all provide a U.S.-style version of the tropics as do South Florida and the Florida Keys, with little worry about traveler's diarrhea.

Danger Signals For the Traveler with IBD

- **High fever and shaking chills.** This could represent a systemic bacterial inflammation requiring intravenous antibiotic therapy.
- **Profuse bloody diarrhea.** This would suggest marked ulceration of the intestine either by a bacterium, parasite, or a major flare-up of colitis.
- **Severe abdominal pain and/or abdominal distension.** This could represent a complication of IBD, especially if associated with severe abdominal tenderness or nausea and vomiting.
- **Dizziness on standing up or an episode of fainting.** This could have several meanings. One is dehydration causing a lowering of blood pressure and requiring intravenous rehydration. Another is "adrenal insufficiency" causing a lowering of blood pressure. An adjustment in steroid dose may be necessary.
- **Scanty, concentrated urine.** With dehydration, the kidneys try to conserve as much fluid as possible. The urine then becomes concentrated (yellow). If fluids cannot be taken by mouth because of associated nausea and vomiting, fluids may have to be provided by intravenous infusion.

If you experience any of these danger signals while traveling, consult a physician immediately.

Questions For Your Physician

Before any trip you will need certain answers from your physician:

1. "What if I have a mild flare-up when I'm away?" Have a written plan for increase in your medication dose and for the use of antispasmodic or antidiarrheal (Lomotil, Imodium, codeine, etc.) medications. What should you do about diet under these circumstances? Again, have a written plan of action regarding dietary modifications.
2. "What if I have a fairly serious flare-up when I'm away?" Obtain a written plan for taking prednisone or antibiotics under these circumstances (e.g. how much and for how many days and in what dosage). Have an adequate supply in case doses need to be raised.
3. "When should I consult a local physician (preferably a gastroenterologist)?" Find out from your physician which are the serious symptoms to look for, but don't ruin your trip by expecting a flare-up to occur.
4. "How about names of physicians who could help me?" Many physicians have colleagues overseas whom they know from their training days or from medical meetings and conferences. Some of them may live and practice in cities you will be visiting. Your doctor can find names and addresses of overseas members of American gastroenterological organizations who will have high levels of skill.

Finally, as you travel, be aware of people around you who could be of help should a medical problem arise. Befriend a physician on your trip and do not be embarrassed about asking for advice or help if the need arises. If a physician is not on your tour, there may be one staying at your hotel. Also bear in mind that other members of the health field, such as nurses, can also be extremely helpful.

For Further Information:

Two useful addressed for the traveler are:

1. The International Association for Medical Assistance to Travelers, (IAMAT), at 736 Center Street, Lewiston, New York 14092, will send (for a donation) a booklet naming doctors in many countries who speak English and will treat IAMAT donors for a set reasonable fee.
2. EuropAssistance, 1333 F. Street, N.W., Washington, D.C. 20004, (202) 347-7113, offers assistance in obtaining medical insurance to handle overseas hospital bills as well as other help to the traveler. Coverage is not available in all states. Previously diagnosed chronic ailments are covered only where there is an emergency situation or complication.

If you become ill when out of the U.S., the nearest U.S. Consulate is a very useful source of information concerning reliable physicians known to the Consulate Staff.

13 How To Be A Hospital Visitor

Introduction

The person who visits an IBD patient in the hospital is capable of offering reassurance and practical information, bolstering the patient's morale, and helping the patient and the patient's family in their emotional response to living with IBD. It is *not* necessary that the hospital visitor also have the disease; family members and friends make excellent visitors.

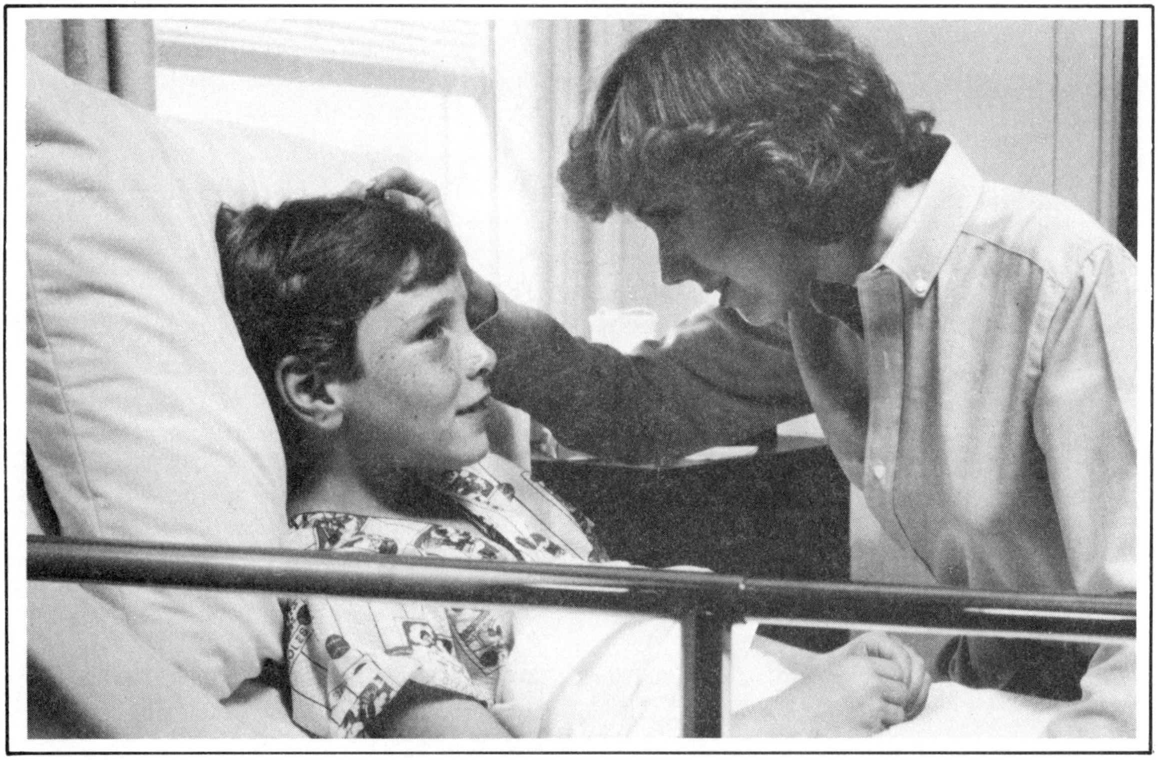

With this in mind, **NFIC's Michigan Chapter** organized a Hospital Visitors Program which operates primarily as a support network for patients with Crohn's disease and ulcerative colitis, their spouses, parents and families. Visitors meet with patients in the hospital in an atmosphere of mutuality of interest and trust. They encourage patients to discuss their physical problems as well as their fears, anxieties and the emotional difficulties associated with IBD.

In this chapter, we present some of the material developed under the Michigan program to illustrate what can be done to lend support to the person with IBD who must be hospitalized.

Some Concerns of IBD Patients in the Hospital

The reaction to the diagnosis of IBD and the ability to face life with a chronic disease vary from one individual to another. To some, adjustment will be a problem, to others a challenge. No matter what the reaction, most patients and their families need a great deal of support right from the time of diagnosis. Support is likely to be most effective when it actively stimulates the person's own inner resources and addresses his/her concerns. There are three major areas of concern common to most IBD patients.

Body Image Issues

Fear of living with a chronic disease is normal. Such thoughts may lead to weeping or depression, or they may be denied. What is the impact of living with IBD on a person's self-image? New patients may refuse to acknowledge the disease, or may hold onto the belief that it is only temporary. Questions may be asked such as: "Is this an emotional disease?" "Am I crazy?" "Will I live or die?" "Will I have to have surgery?" "How will I look?" "Will I be able to have sex?" "Will I ever be normal again?"

There are times when people must have the opportunity to express or deny their feelings about the changes in their bodies or their self-image. Expression of negative feelings is a way to release the tension and anxiety and is not inappropriate in a crisis situation. Temporary denial is a useful mechanism which allows people to face reality gradually.

Hospital patients must not feel contradicted by their visitors, but they do need to learn from them about reality. They need to find out that others have felt as they do, that others have learned to deal with negative feelings, have overcome them and that in time they will do so, too.

Issues of Control

There are those who fear that they may never again be in control of their own lives. They may want others to assume physical care and may consider themselves invalids, unable to resume usual daily activities. Questions may be asked such as: "How will my medication affect me?" "How did it affect you?" "What about bathrooms?" "What about traveling?" "What about work?"

If the visitor has IBD and has maintained his or her activities, this is frequently persuasive evidence that the job can be done and may help to turn the tide of apprehension. Just seeing another person with the same illness functioning and looking well gives them hope. Patients need to be reassured that maintaining their lifestyle is possible.

Relationships with Others

A third concern is the hospitalized patient's perception of his/her relationships with others. Like many others with chronic problems, they may fear that their social role may have changed, that others may not accept them as in the past. They may be worried about sexuality (both interpersonal and physical) and whether close relationships will be possible. Going to work may be a major source of worry. How to tell others may be troublesome. *Should* they tell others? How will the disease affect spouse, friends, family, children, careers, marriage, having children?

The visitor must let the patient know that these are matters that not only can be but *should* be discussed. The visitor is in an ideal position to demonstrate to patients that their social selves need not be changed. Visitors must always bear in mind that it takes time to work through feelings associated with crisis and that they cannot be glossed over. On the other hand, if a patient seems to cling to negative feelings and ideas, the help of a professional person is probably indicated.

Remember, there is a fine line between practical information based on the visitor's experience and the giving of medical advice. The visitor must be vigilant not to cross that line!

Making the Visit

The approach to the hospital patient varies from person to person and is also affected by the situation. The questions to be considered are: What is the hospital patient facing at this time? What help can I give now? First visits may need to be short to avoid tiring the patient. Regardless of when the first visit is made, the fundamental purposes remain the same:

- To let the patient know that a normal life is possible and that he/she is not alone.
- To allow the patient to express his/her feelings.
- To assure the patient of available help.
- To give comfort to patient and family.

Techniques for the Successful Visitor

To assure privacy if the patient is not in a single room, ask if he/she would like the curtain drawn. If there are other visitors, ask the patient if he/she wishes to speak to you alone or with others present, or whether you should come back at a later time. Sit where the patient can see you easily without turning his/her head. When you sit, you are on the same level, and communication may come more easily.

Encourage the patient to ask questions. Answer the questions tactfully and honestly. If you don't know the answer, say so. Above all, don't dwell on *your* medical history and/or surgery. This visit belongs to the patient.

Accept any emotional responses. If the person is angry or feels like crying, don't stop him/her. Accepting feelings will usually make you both feel closer. Remember that nonverbal communication is meaningful. A touch or a smile may do far more than the spoken word.

Keep these important points in mind:

- Stress normal life, physical and social activities.
- Answer all questions honestly and briefly, with limited detail.
- Use active listening skills (See material in this chapter).
- Refer all medical and surgical questions to medical personnel.
- Assure the patient of your assistance.
- Acquaint the patient with the NFIC and the local chapter but do not solicit membership.
- Leave appropriate NFIC literature if the person wishes it. Invite him/her to next NFIC education meeting.

Active Listening: A Useful Visiting Technique

In communication, nothing takes the place of a healthy instinct. Sometimes we know just what to say and do. But to rely on it totally would be like sailing without a compass. Over the years, visiting techniques have been developed which have proven very helpful. They should be studied and put into practice. The techniques of active listening, if learned and practiced, will enable you to become an effective visitor even if your instinct should fail you momentarily.

Since a major purpose of active listening is to understand what a person is thinking and feeling, we must listen to the words that are spoken, to the way they are spoken, and to note the expression that accompanies them. We all have experienced situations in which what is said and how it comes across are not in harmony. When a person is under stress, such discrepancies are not uncommon. You will need to be very attentive so that you will not miss what the patient is trying to communicate.

Another purpose of active listening is to help another person. In the process of explaining his/her thoughts and feelings to you, the person often comes to better understand the problem at hand. When we listen and respond actively, we are structuring an atmosphere which provides opportunities for the patient to understand himself or herself better and to take responsibility for altering the situation.

Here are some examples of how active listening may be used in a conversation:

Technique	Listener's Response
Show an interest in what the person is saying.	"I see,...oh,...uh-huh..."
Encourage the individual to expand on the problem or question.	"Yes, go on...tell me more..."
Help the individual clarify the problem in his/her own thinking.	"Then the problem, *as you* see it, is..."
Help the individual hear what he/she said in the way it sounded to you.	"This is *your* situation then,...and I heard *you* saying that..."
Identify key ideas in a long statement.	"Your main point is...*you* feel that..."
Respond to the person's feelings as well as to his words.	"I guess *you* feel strongly that..."
Allow silence.	Non-verbal behavior will let the patient know you are with him/her; use eye contact, posture.

Do's and Don'ts of Hospital Visiting

DO:

- Make the visit as promised and in a timely manner.
- Adhere to the purpose of the visit.
- Practice appropriate hospital etiquette.
- Use active listening skills.
- Be friendly, tactful, considerate and compassionate.
- Be neat and clean in dress and appearance.
- Leave NFIC literature if patients wish it.

DON'T:

- Give medical advice.
- Explain your own life story.
- Contradict physician or any other member of health care team.
- Frighten the patient or family members.
- Solicit membership in NFIC.
- Overtire patient.
- Sit on bed.
- Smoke, chew gum or wear perfume during the visit.
- Interfere with hospital routine.
- Interfere with family interaction.

For Further Information...

Michigan Chapter
National Foundation for Ileitis and Colitis
Suite 238
Southfield, MI 48075
313-424-8656 or 313-424-8657

14

Organizing A Self-Help Group For People With IBD

Introduction: What is Self-Help?

"Self-help" means more than just helping yourself. In practice, it has come to mean people with a mutual interest who come together to be helped in a support situation, and who remain to help others. The self-help movement has been described as one of the major national trends of the past decade, and there are in existence today over 500,000 self-help or mutual support groups. There are 25 Self-Help Clearinghouses across the country helping to refer people to groups and training new group leaders. Why has this phenomenon grown so rapidly?

In 1978, President Carter's Commission on Mental Health reported that there were very few support services available to help people who were not acutely ill. These people, many of whom were suffering from chronic illnesses or shared a mutual need or handicap, were simply not receiving sufficient attention from the organized mental health establishment. Self-help groups have been able to fill this gap in human services left by mental health budget cuts. Self-help groups are also a partial solution to the high mobility of today's society and often function as "extended family" in giving social support. These groups operate on the simple premise that helping someone else—something with which we all have experience—makes us feel better. And when we feel better, we can usually cope better.

What Self-Help is Not

Self-help groups are not therapy groups led by professionals. Neither are they a substitute for professional therapy when that is what is needed. Although a self-help group may work closely with a professional such as a psychologist or social worker, the group relies on its members or "peers" for support. Members of a group should at some time be both "helper" and "helped" in order for the group to succeed.

In their book, *Self-Help in the Human Services,* Alan Gartner and Frank Riessman list some characteristics which they consider essential to any kind of self-help group and which distinguish them from other types of groups:

- Self-help groups always involve face-to-face interactions.
- The origin of self-help groups is usually spontaneous (not set up by some outside group).
- Personal participation is an extremely important ingredient.
- The members agree on and engage in some actions.
- Typically the groups start from a condition of powerlessness.
- The group fills the needs for a reference group, a point of connection and identification with others, a base for activity, and a source of ego reinforcement.

Self-Help Groups and IBD

Crohn's disease and ulcerative colitis are the type of medical condition for which self-help or mutual support groups can be extremely beneficial. People with IBD often feel terribly isolated, as though there is no one who *really* understands what they are going through. Symptoms like chronic pain, weakness, diarrhea and bleeding are not easily discussed, even among friends and family members. Few outsiders can appreciate the extreme anxiety associated with the need to be near to a bathroom which is experienced by many people with IBD. For many, their participation in support groups may be the first time they have ever met and talked with another person with Crohn's disease or ulcerative colitis and shared their anxieties and problems in coping with IBD.

Many chapters of the National Foundation for Ileitis and Colitis have formed successful self-help or mutual support groups. These include groups for patients only, parent groups, singles or couples groups, and groups of teenagers. Some chapters are led by volunteer lay members of the group, others use psychologists or social workers as consultants. A directory of NFIC chapters appears in the Appendix of this book. If there is no NFIC chapter or IBD support group in your area, this information should help you to take the first steps necessary to start a group and to keep it going.

Getting Started

"Self-help doesn't start until you find at least one other person with whom to share."[1]

The first thing you have to do is to identify other people with IBD who would benefit from a support group. Obviously, this is easier to do if you belong to a local NFIC chapter and can work within the chapter framework, using the chapter structure to help with publicity, mailings, meeting space, etc. If there is not yet an NFIC chapter in your area to help you, you can put up notices on the bulletin boards of local hospitals or try to get referrals from gastroenterologists and/or internists in your area. Notices in newspapers and on radio can also be used. It is essential to find a core of interested people with whom to share the initial burden of organizing so that you will not have to do it alone.

The core group needs to decide the *goals* of the group to be formed, based on the target population (IBD patients and their families), and the *methods* it will use to accomplish these goals. It isn't enough that all members have a particular disease–IBD–in common. It's essential to discuss the reasons why this IBD support group is being established and what an IBD support group might hope to accomplish. Here are some primary group goals other IBD support groups have listed:

- Promote fellowship and dispel sense of isolation.
- Give support and encouragement to others.
- Share coping strategies.
- Release negative feelings like guilt.
- Strengthen self-esteem.
- Concentrate on abilities, not disabilities.
- Exchange ideas and resources.
- Meet new friends.

Here are some questions the core group might then ask itself:

- What are the support needs of IBD patients in our community?
- How should we choose a group format that will satisfy those needs?
- How do we create a "safe" and comfortable location for sharing needs and promoting interaction so people stay connected to the group?
- Should we use professionals as consultants?
- How do we become good lay leaders and train others?
- Should we have a mixed group (patients, spouses, parents) or should there be separate groups?
- Should there be a fee charged?
- How can we win support from the medical community?
- How can we keep the group interested and involved once it has started?

Once you have discussed and resolved these questions, you are ready to examine the types of self-help groups and decide which one might be best for your community.

1. Andy Humm: *How to organize a Self-Help Group:* New York City Self-Help Clearinghouse, 1979.

Models of Self-Help Groups

Three group models are discussed here. Each model has advantages and disadvantages which may make it more or less appealing to your group.

The ***Indigenously-led group*** is a small informal group or "rap" session led by a lay person who may share the same condition or experience —in this case inflammatory bowel disease—with other members of the group. Since the leader is not a trained professional, and may occasionally suffer from "burn-out" or ill health, a co-leader is often advisable. Indigenously-led groups generally meet on a regular basis, weekly or twice a month, either in a meeting place or in someone's home. The frequency of meeting helps cement a feeling of trust and confidentiality in the group. Many of these groups ask for a small donation to cover the costs of publicity, phone calls, refreshments, etc. Because of their intimate nature, these groups may start small, sometimes with as few as three or four interested people. It takes courage for some people to begin to talk about personal problems in a group situation. For such people, simply knowing the group exists, and that they *could* come if they wished, is often comfort enough. In time, they will hopefully join the group.

Professionally-led groups ask the guidance of a mental health professional such as a psychologist or social worker as either group leader, group facilitator, or consultant. In these groups, the professional is usually selected because of his/her skill and experience in group dynamics and *not* because of expertise in a particular disease or condition. Group members would understand far better than the professional what it's like to live with a chronic disease like IBD. For this reason, it is important for the core group itself to decide the extent of the professional's participation in the group. Some professionals could be used simply to get a group started and running, while others could be used to guide discussion in the group.

Lecture/discussion groups use an outside expert, or panel of experts—physicians, nurses, pharmacists or other professionals—to impart information, after which the meeting format moves either to a question and answer session or a group discussion or several small group discussions of what was presented at the lecture. While this format may be ideal for rural areas where there is no NFIC chapter or where education meetings are fewer and travel may be difficult, it does not lend itself to easy discussion between peers. Given the formal arrangement of chairs, often in classroom style, it is not easy to break out of the passive role of listener and become an active participant in a discussion. For many, the presence of an "expert" can also be quite inhibiting.

As you can see, in order to decide among these group models, your core group must first decide whether its *real* goal is to foster support relationships *or* to impart information about IBD. This is a crucial distinction because transition from a lecture/discussion format to an informal support group is extremely difficult. Once you have chosen the model which best suits your core group's needs, your thinking process should look something like this schematic diagram:

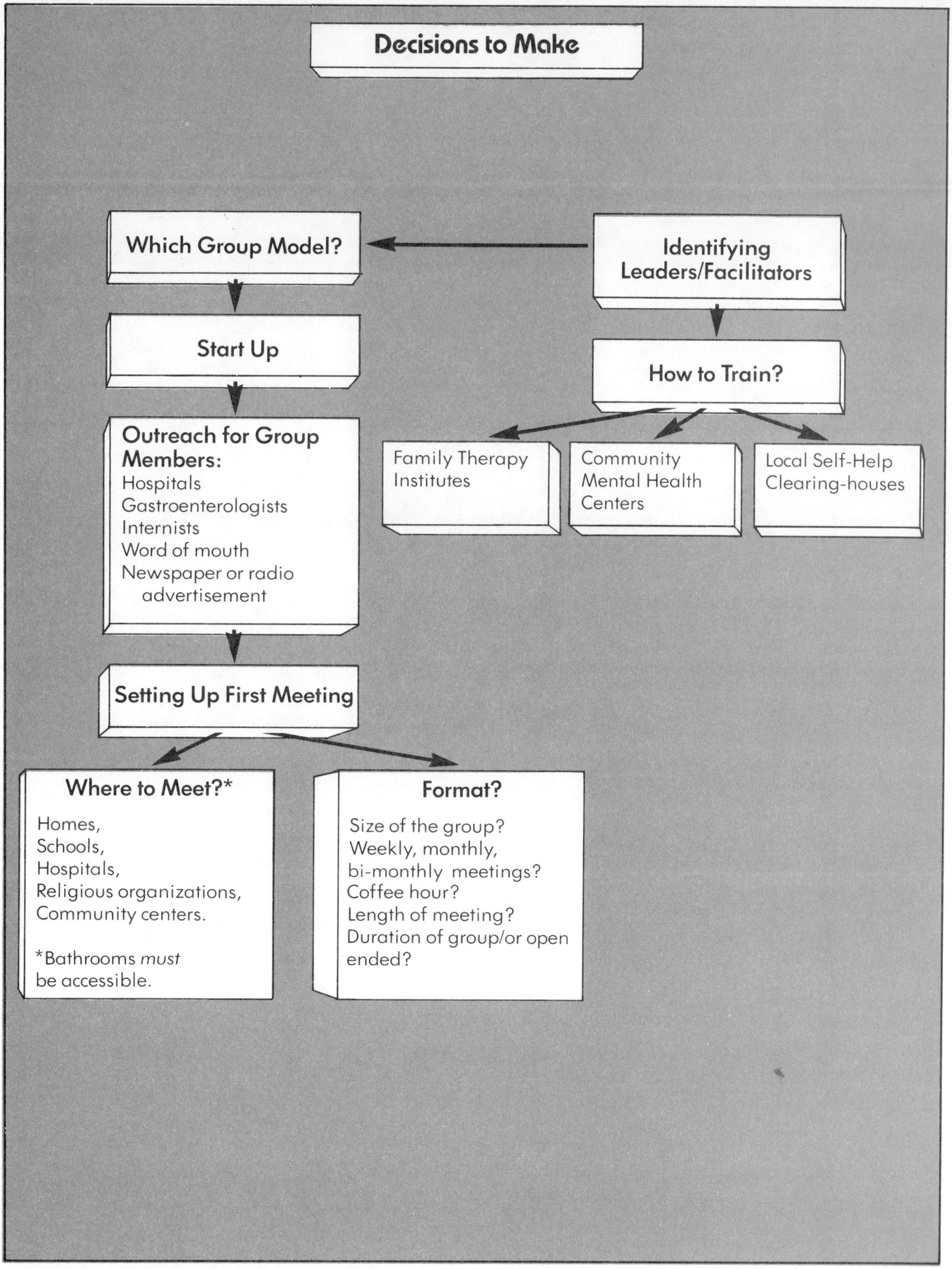
Decisions to Make
Which Group Model?
Identifying Leaders/Facilitators
Start Up
How to Train?
Family Therapy Institutes
Community Mental Health Centers
Local Self-Help Clearing-houses
Outreach for Group Members:
Hospitals
Gastroenterologists
Internists
Word of mouth
Newspaper or radio advertisement
Setting Up First Meeting
Where to Meet?*
Homes,
Schools,
Hospitals,
Religious organizations,
Community centers.
*Bathrooms *must* be accessible.
Format?
Size of the group?
Weekly, monthly, bi-monthly meetings?
Coffee hour?
Length of meeting?
Duration of group/or open ended?

Winning Over the Physicians

Occasionally, the physician or a group of physicians can become an obstacle to setting up a self-help program for IBD patients and their families. Some physicians resist the self-help movement perhaps because they see it as a threat to the doctor-patient relationship. Others misunderstand the role of self-help and assume it is "psychotherapy" performed by amateurs. The root of the problem, as one physician puts it, is that "we doctors are trained to think of ourselves as healers and of patients as sufferers. We haven't thought of support organizations as a place to turn to help patients." This physician only became aware of the power of self-help when "my patients told me what a help it was for them to talk to other patients in the waiting room who had the same problem." When actually exposed to self-help and support groups and what they can do for their patients, most physicians eventually become enthusiastic supporters.

What Other Physicians Have Said About Self-Help

- "Sometimes patients hesitate to ask physicians about non-medical aspects of the disease, such as family reactions to the affected member, job and insurance problems, physician-patient relationships, sexual problems and emotional difficulties. Although most physicians are glad to handle these questions, patients may feel more comfortable talking with others who have experienced the same problems."
- "Articulate, empathetic patients who counsel new patients make the journey easier for both the patient and the physician. Uncounseled, unassisted, the patient is often lost, bewildered, and depressed, demanding continuous attention and time from the physician, nurses, and social workers. But with the aid of someone who has been there, the patient demands less of the physician concerning family and emotional problems that the physician may not be trained to handle."

Setting the Stage for the First Meeting

Regardless of which group model you have chosen, certain practical issues must be addressed *before* the date of the first meeting. These include:

1. ***Size of the group:*** While a discussion group can be any size, there is more opportunity for participation and sharing of experiences if the group has between six and ten people. If, for example, in the lecture/discussion model, a large group has just listened to a lecture presentation, smaller groups can be broken out of the large group to give everyone a chance to participate and to prevent domination of discussion by the more vocal group members.

2. ***Seating and atmosphere:*** Whenever possible, arrange chairs in a circle to let each member feel like an equal participant. Avoid "classroom style" set-ups which discourage eye contact. Paying attention to details such as comfortable chairs, room temperature and quiet surroundings will contribute to the success of the meeting. You may want to let the group decide if it wants to serve coffee and refreshments.

3. ***Confidentiality:*** Because group members will be sharing sensitive information about their illness or that of a loved one, all members should mutually agree that what is said in the group remains confidential.

4. ***Duration of the group:*** The core group should decide in advance how long each session should be (one and a half to two hours is suggested), how often to meet, and whether the group will be time limited to six or eight weeks or open-ended. Time limited groups work well in cities where public transportation is available, but do not generally incorporate new members into the group after a week or two. Open-ended groups are better in areas where members are traveling from a distance and may have to miss several meetings. They also have the advantage of allowing members to enter and leave the group.

Group Leadership

If your core group has chosen the indigenously-led group model, it is likely that one or more of you will become the group's first leaders or facilitators. Since leadership is a function or a process and not a person, you need not have great charismatic appeal or speaking ability to become an effective leader. What skills are helpful in facilitating or leading group discussion? The following list of skills probably includes many which you and your core group members already possess:

- Listening actively to what is being said.
- Keeping discussion moving and group members on topic.
- Encouraging participation by all group members.
- Accepting feelings as OK.
- Suggesting ways to solve a problem.
- Summarizing what has been said.
- Clarifying the direction of discussion.

Many successful group leaders begin a discussion by sharing with the group their personal reasons for becoming involved. This could take the form of a description of their reaction to having IBD or to being the spouse or parent of a person with IBD. Use of the words "I" or "me" is very important at this stage and throughout the group process because it helps the group to see that your participation is real. Personalizing your experience also helps the group to understand your reasons for wanting to be a group leader and serves as a stimulus for others to begin talking about themselves.

Skills for Group Leadership

As a group leader, you have developed or will need to develop specific skills to facilitate discussion. Some of these skills are listed below:

1. ***Listen actively.*** In any discussion, it is easy to let your attention wander. As group leader/facilitator, you should listen as much to *how* things are said as to *what* is being said. You should observe the atmosphere in the room, e.g. whether people are looking at each other, what non-verbal clues your group members are giving you. As leader, you may actually do less talking than anyone else in the group in order to give all group members the opportunity to talk and to share their experiences.

2. ***Learn to ask open-ended questions.*** Phrase questions with words like "How did that make you feel?" or "What do others feel about that?" or "Does anyone else want to comment?" Ask questions that will open discussion, not close it. Don't ask leading questions which manipulate others. Instead of asking, "Don't you think this was a great meeting?," ask "What did you think of the meeting?"

3. ***Learn to use "I" statements.*** When you are making a contribution to the discussion, don't generalize your feelings to the whole group. Identify your feelings as your own by using the words "I" and "me." Express yourself openly and honestly. As leader, it is difficult to expect people to share their feelings if you won't share yours.

4. ***Respond to the feelings expressed by others.*** Accept the feelings of others as valid. Don't interpret or be judgmental; don't give evaluations or ask why someone feels the way they do. Direct "why" questions make people feel uncomfortable and defensive.

5. ***Allow the group members to help.*** You want members of the group to feel it is *their* group, not your group. By allowing group members to support each other by offering practical suggestions or by relating their own personal experience, you encourage them to invest in the group and stay involved.

What to Talk About?

After the group is underway and members are beginning to get to know each other, new group leaders worry that there might not be enough to talk about in group sessions, or that there may be long, uncomfortable silences. Although experience with IBD support groups has shown that there is more than enough to talk about, some new leaders may feel more comfortable with a list of possible topics to introduce. The following topics have been used by support groups in some NFIC chapters; the questions can be used to help stimulate discussion.

1. ***Reaction to Having a Chronic Illness:*** What does it feel like to find out, perhaps half-way through life, that you have a chronic illness? How did you find out, what were your early symptoms? Did you get the right diagnosis the first time?

2. ***Reaction of Friends and Family:*** Who is your support system? Is it a parent, spouse, sibling, friend? How did your support system react when you were first diagnosed? Were you given erroneous advice from friends and well-wishers about the nature of your illness? (Many group members may have been told their disease was due to stress or poor eating habits, etc.) Is it easy to ask for help when you need it? How does your support system react to long bouts or flare-ups?

3. ***Impact of IBD on Lifestyle:*** Can you work, go to school, take vacation, go out with friends? Have you missed work days or classes? How have the teachers or employers reacted to your illness? Have there been good or bad experiences to share along these lines? If you are single, can you have a social life that is normal? Are there certain precautions you take if you know you will be taking a long car ride not knowing where the next bathroom may be? Is your life sometimes dependent on where the bathroom is? Can you be open about that need, or must it be a secret?

4. ***Dealing with Your Physician:*** Is your doctor available to you? Does he answer all your questions? Do you feel he may be holding information back? Has he told you about the possible side-effects of your medication? Does he spend time with you on the phone?

5. ***Feelings About Medical Treatment:*** How do you feel about surgery, tests, having to take medications such as prednisone? What are the effects of prednisone on your mood, your appearance, the way you feel about yourself? How do you feel about trying new medications?

6. ***Feelings About Sex:*** Do you have fears about something happening during sexual intercourse (particularly with single people), fears of being unattractive, fears about having children? How open can you be with a prospective mate without scaring him/her off? How to explain the side-effects of medication to a friend or mate?

7. ***Using the Illness:*** Is it possible to use your illness to get attention or pity? Is it a way to cop out when necessary? Do sick youngsters get more attention from their parents? How does that create problems in the family? When is psychotherapy a good idea?

8. ***Sharing Coping Strategies:*** Is it a good idea to carry an extra change of underwear at all times, or a portable toilet in the car, or to check ahead to find where the bathrooms are located? Should you talk to teachers on behalf of a child to make sure of immediate access to toilet facilities, etc.?

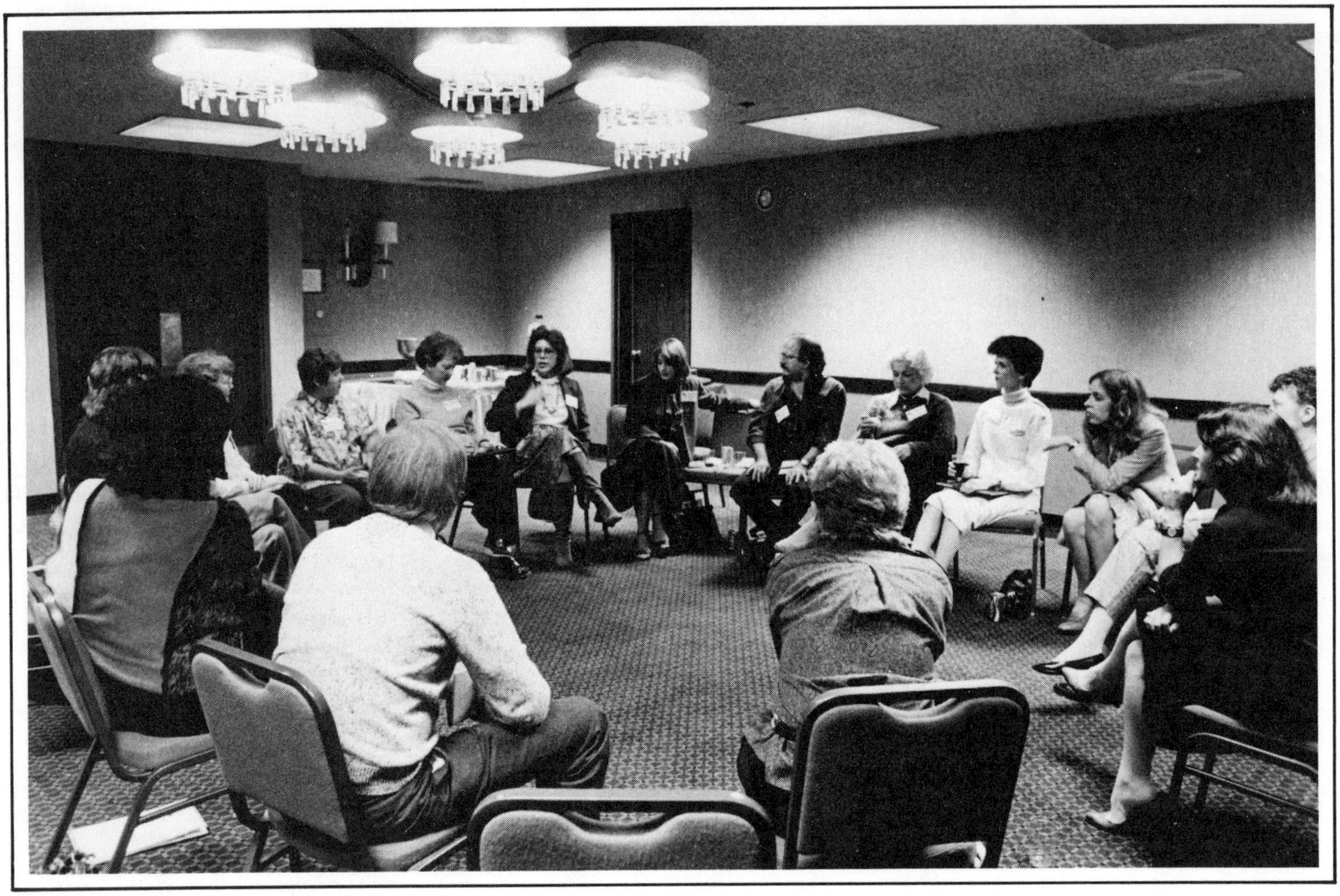

Introducing a Topic

While the use of structured discussion topics is optional and can often prevent repetition and boredom, some group members may resent being told what to discuss. Rather than introduce a topic directly, the group leader may begin by expressing his/her feelings on a particular subject. For example, "When I was first diagnosed, I had many feelings–anger, frustration, isolation. I was wondering if anyone else has experienced these feelings?" This approach invites the expression of feelings from other members of the group and introduces a topic for discussion in a way that is non-threatening and non-authoritarian.

It is important to remember that as group leader you have a dual role: You must direct the discussion and try to keep the group on topic, but you are also a member of the group and must share your experiences. By expressing these experiences in a "directive" way, you model the responses of the other group members. You need only strike the spark; you do not need to nurture the group continually.

Group Maintenance

The life of a group is never static–it has peaks and valleys. If it is an open-ended group, new people are entering as other group members leave. Some groups adopt a "buddy" system to make new members feel at home. Occasionally, members may be hospitalized with a relapse and may need more support from the group. Other members may out grow their need for support as they begin to feel stronger. One way to determine if your group's needs are being met is to administer a questionnaire at the end of a time-limited group, or to those leaving an open-ended group. (See appendix to this chapter.)

Group leaders, too, have their ups and downs. It is possible to become tired, "burned-out" or experience a flare-up of their illness. Or they may have invested too many emotions in the success of the group and may become overburdened and depressed. The use of co-leaders can forestall this problem. It is also important to have a mechanism in place to train and/or recruit new group leaders from within the group itself. Local community mental health centers and self-help clearinghouses are an excellent resource for training in group leadership. (A listing of self-help clearinghouses in the U.S. appears as an appendix to this chapter.)

It is important to remember that if your group disbands, as many groups do, it may be a sign that the group has been successful and no longer needs to exist. Remember that the self-help and support that began in the group continues between individuals long afterward.

For Further Information...

Hill, Karen: *Helping You Helps Me: A Guide Book for Self-Help Groups.* Ottawa: Canadian Council on Social Development.
Humm, Andy: *How to Organize a Self-Help Group,* New York; New York City Self-Help Clearinghouse, 1979.
Manber, Malcolm M: "Patient support groups: a natural resource for physicians," *Medical World News,* December 10, 1984.

Self-Help Group Questionnaire

In order for us to continue to evaluate the success of the Self-Help program, we would appreciate your answering the following questionnaire as completely as possible, and returning it to the Chapter office. You may sign it if you wish. Your aswers will remain confidential. Thank you for your help with this important project.

PART I

1. How did you hear of the Self-Help program? ______
2. Did your group meet in the geographical location of your choice?
   ☐ yes ☐ no If not, which location would you have preferred? ______
3. What was the approximate number of participants? ______
   Would you have preferred it to be larger or smaller? ______
4. What was the make-up of your group (i.e., patients, parents, young adults)? Was the make-up satisfactory to you? If not, how would you have preferred it? ______
5. What was your reaction to the length of the session? Was it long enough? Do you feel there was sufficient time to cover the subject matter? ______
6. Would you be interested in becoming a group leader? ______
7. Would you join another group at a future time? ______

PART II

1. Can you describe your expectations in joining a Self-Help group? ______
2. Would you say that these expectations were realized? ______
3. Where there any unexpected benefits derived from the experience? ______
4. What were your reactions to the other members in your group? ______
5. What was your reaction to the group leader(s)? ______
6. Were there any aspects of the discussion which you found disturbing? ______
7. Were there any subjects which you felt should be included and were not? ______
8. Do you feel this program is meaningful to the over-all goals of the NFIC? How? ______
9. Would you please summarize your feelings about the total experience? ______

Name: ______ (not required)

North Eastern and Middle Atlantic States:

New York:

New York City Self-Help Clearinghouse
Frances J. Dory, Executive Director
186 Joralemon Street
Brooklyn, New York 11201
(718) 852-4290
Services 5 boroughs of New York City

Brooklyn Self-Help Clearinghouse
Heights and Hill Mental Health Service
Carol Berkvist, CSS Coordinator
50 Court Street
Brooklyn, New York 11201
(718) 834-7341
Services Kings County

Long Island Self-Help Action Center
New York Institute of Technology
Audrey Leif, Coordinator
Commack College Center
6350 Jericho Turnpike
Commack, New York 11725
(516) 499-8800
Services Nassau and Suffolk Counties

Westchester Self-Help Clearinghouse
Leslie Borck, Ph.D., Director
Westchester Community College
Academic Arts Building
75 Grasslands Road
Valhalla, New York 10595
(914) 347-3620
Services Westchester County

National Self-Help Clearinghouse
Frank Riessman, Ph.D., Director
City University of New York
33 West 42nd Street
New York City, New York 10036
(212) 840-1259

New Jersey:

New Jersey Self-Help Clearinghouse
Edward J. Madera, Director
St. Clare's Hospital CMHC
Denville, New Jersey 07834
(201) 625-7101 out of state
(800) FOR-MASH in state callers

Connecticut:

Connecticut Self-Help/Mutual Support Network
Vicki Spiro Smith, Coordinator
Consultation Center
19 Howe Street
New Haven, Connecticut 06511
(203) 789-7645

Pennsylvania:

Philadelphia Self-Help Clearinghouse
Debby Tolson, Director
John F. Kennedy CMHC
112 North Broad Street
Philadelphia, Pennsylvania 19102
(215) 568-0890 ext. 266

Self-Help Information and Networking Exchange (SHINE)
Arlene Hopkins, Director
Voluntary Action Center of NE Pennsylvania
200 Adams Avenue
Scranton, PA 18503
(717) 961-1234

District of Columbia:

Greater Washington Self-Help Coalition
(Washington, D.C., Northern Virginia, and Southern Maryland)
Linda Figuerosa, Coordinator
Mental Health Association of Northern Virginia
100 North Washington Street Suite 232
Falls Church, Virginia 22046
(703) 536-4100

Midwestern and Great Lakes States:

Illinois:

Self-Help Center, Inc.
Leonard D. Borman, Ph.D., Director
1600 Dodge Center, Suite S122
Evanston, Illinois 60201
(312) 828-0470

Michigan:
Berrien County Self-Help Clearinghouse
Rob Hess and Charles Livingston, Coordinators
Riverwood Community Mental Health Center
2681 Morton Avenue
St. Joseph, Michigan 49085
(616) 642-4060

Kansas:
Sedgwick County Self-Help Clearinghouse
Evelyn Middlestadt, M.S.W. Coordinator
3428 East Central
Wichita, Kansas 62708
(316) 686-1205

Minnesota:
Minnesota Mutual Help Resource Center
Gloria Johnson, Information Specialist
Wilder Foundation Community Care Unit
919 Lafond Avenue
St. Paul, Minnesota 55104
(612) 642-4060

Nebraska:
Self-Help Information Services
Barbara Fox, Director
1601 Euclid Avenue
Lincoln, Nebraska 68502
(402) 476-6998

Wisconsin:
Mutual Aid Self-Help Association (MASHA)
Lu Mallory, President
1610 East Newport Avenue
Milwaukee, Wisconsin 53211
(414) 461-1466

Southwest:

Texas:
Mental Health Association of Dallas County
Carol Madison, Staff Associate
2500 Maple Avenue
Dallas, Texas 75201
(214) 748-7825

Far West:

California:
California Self-Help Center
Carol Eisman, Public Education Specialist
UCLA
405 Hilgard Avenue
Los Angeles, California 90024
(213) 825-1799

Mental Health Association of Merced County
Geri Stewart, Coordinator
Merced, California 95341
(209) 723-8861

Self-Help Network
Mental Health Association of Santa Maria
P.O. Box 104
Santa Maria, California 934
(805) 922-2165

San Francisco Self-Help Clearinghouse
Ruth Tabbits, Director
Mental Health Association of San Francisco
2398 Pine Street
San Francisco, California 94115
(415) 921-4401

Mental Health Association of Sacramento
Janice Manfred, Coordinator
5370 Elvas Avenue
Sacramento, California 95819
(916) 456-2070

San Diego Self-Help Clearinghouse
Ellen Murphy, Director
1172 Morena Boulevard
San Diego, California 92103

Oregon
Tri- County Community Council
(503) 222-5555

If a self-help resource center is not listed in your area, try contacting the local community council, mental health association or help-line/hotline switchboard. These organizations often have lists of self-help groups.

III

Knowing Your Rights

15

Obtaining And Understanding Your Medical Records

Anyone familiar with the rise of consumerism in the health field would argue that the appetite of the American public for medical information is increasing dramatically. Consumer groups are compiling physician directories and pushing for increased health awareness among all sectors of the population. A glance at the health book section in any book store reveals a flood of new titles on every aspect of health and disease. This new awareness also takes the form of an intense desire for control over information about the health care we are receiving and paying for. Yet the one document which is likely to contain the greatest amount of information pertinent to our personal health–the medical record–often remains inaccessible. This chapter will explain what is contained in the medical record, why it is important for the person with IBD to have access to that record (or to parts of it), and how to go about obtaining it.

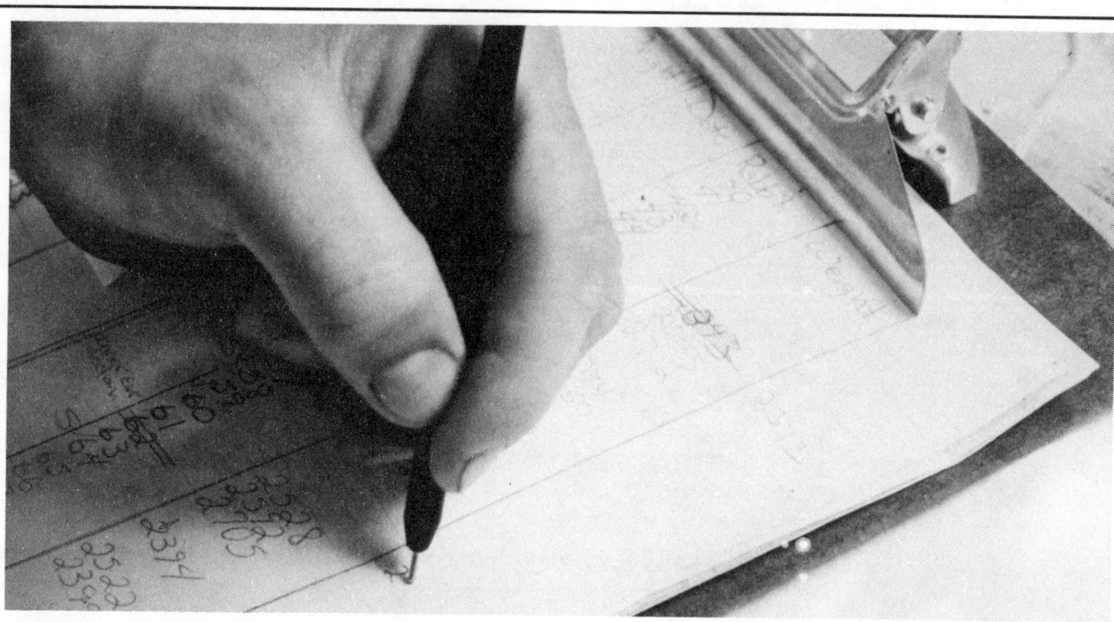

What is in Your Hospital Medical Record?

Your hospital medical record contains documentation about why you were admitted to the hospital, what laboratory tests and diagnostic procedures were performed while you were there, what were the results, and what was your progress (or lack of it) during the hospital stay. This record is both a valuable communication tool between the members of the health care team who care for you and an important legal document of the care you have received while in the hospital. Your record begins to accumulate forms from the moment you enter the admitting office and are assigned a unit number; information is added to your record until, and even after, you leave the hospital. The "chart," as it is called by hospital personnel, is kept at the nurses' station on your unit, and all hospital personnel who participate in your care are required to make entries regarding your treatment. After you are discharged, your record is sent to the medical record department of the hospital. When all forms are completed and signed, your record is then filed under the unit number assigned to you at admission. Subsequent hospital admissions will use this same unit number, so that information on multiple hospitalizations is bound together in one record.

The Parts of Your Hospital Record

The following forms are standard parts of all hospital medical records:

face sheet—contains admitting and billing information (name, address, employer, insurance carrier), admitting diagnosis. Final diagnosis is added upon discharge.

admission note—records your condition on admission, including results of recent tests.

history and physical examination—contains your complete medical history as told to the admitting resident, as well as results of physical examination.

graphic record—a record of your temperature, pulse, respiration and blood pressure while in the hospital.

progress notes—a daily record of your progress, test results, etc. by the professionals who care for you.

doctor's order sheets—a record of the medications ordered for you by your physicians.

x-ray reports—results of diagnostic x-rays.

laboratory reports—results of various tests.

nursing notes, admitting forms and medication record—separate entries made by the nursing staff.

operative report—a complete record of any operation dictated by the surgeon after surgery.

pathology report—results of examination of any tissues removed from your body at operation or biopsy.

discharge summary—a summary dictated by your physician during or after the hospital stay, including any tests or operations performed, laboratory data, your condition on discharge, and plans for your follow-up care.

Users of the Medical Record

The medical record is legally the property of the hospital, and whether or not you have the right to see or have a copy of your medical record depends on what laws have been passed in your state. At the same time, the *information* contained in the record is confidential in nature and is "owned" by the patient. For this reason, anyone admitted to a hospital must sign a release authorizing the hospital to permit inspection of the record by insurance companies, Blue Cross, or government payers (Medicare, Medicaid) in order to verify the care that has been rendered. In addition, the broad wording of most release-of-information authorizations permits access to your record by law enforcement agencies, schools, social service agencies, hospital risk managers, and by medical researchers on the hospital staff. Moreover, insurance companies pool the information obtained from claims review in a large computerized data bank of which most people are totally unaware. Hospital patients have asked, logically, how they can possibly make an informed decision to authorize the use of their records by third parties when they themselves have not seen those records and have no idea what they contain.

The Importance of Access

In these days of increased participation by people in their own health care, the arguments favoring patient access to the medical record are stronger than ever. This is especially true for persons with a chronic illness such as IBD. In the past, members of the medical profession have sought to prevent patient access to this information, claiming that patients could not possibly understand their charts. Unfortunately, some doctors interpret these requests from their patients as a loss of trust rather than as a desire to learn more about their conditions. Recently, however, the American Hospital Association, in a reversal of its earlier position, has taken a stand supporting the right of patients to obtain complete medical information from doctors, provided they will not be harmed medically by what they read.

Access to pertinent medical record information means that "patients" can start acting more like "consumers" in selecting the best health care available to them and avoiding unnecessary and costly procedures.

People have little to lose and a lot to gain from seeing all or part of their hospital records. First, there is the obvious sense of relief at having the secrecy removed from the record, together with the more open physician-patient partnership which is likely to result. Access to written records also increases a person's sense of responsibility in making important health care decisions. Possession of at least a part of the record, such as the Discharge Summary, Operative Report, Endoscopy

Report, Pathology Report, and the results and actual copies of recent x-rays, is helpful in assuring continuity of care when a person changes physicians, moves to another part of the country, or is in an emergency situation requiring immediate access to medical information. Access to pertinent medical record information means that "patients" can start acting more like "consumers" in selecting the best health care available to them and avoiding unnecessary and costly procedures.

Gaining Access to Your Records

Whether or not you have legal access to your hospital records depends upon where you live. Since the hospital is the legal owner of the record, right to access can be granted only by state laws (statutes) or by case law in a particular state. State laws vary greatly as to the types of records covered (i.e. hospital records or doctors' office records), who has access to those records (i.e. patient, attorney or physician), and the form of access (i.e. whether a patient is entitled to see or copy the record, or is entitled to a summary only).

Fifteen states now provide for some sort of patient access (direct or indirect) to both hospital and doctor's records (Alaska, California, Colorado, Florida, Hawaii, Illinois, Louisiana, Michigan, Minnesota, Nevada, Oklahoma, Oregon, Utah, Virginia and Wisconsin). Nine other states grant access to hospital records only (Connecticut, Indiana, Maine, Massachusetts, Mississippi, Nebraska, New Jersey, South Dakota and Tennessee), and New York State has a law granting access to doctor's records only. This leaves about half the states with no statutes at all.

To check on your right to access in your state, you should write or call the Public Citizen Health Research Group, 2000 P Street, N.W., Washington, D.C. 20036. Remember that pending legislation may have been passed since the publication of this list. To find out if there are any medical record access bills pending in your state, write to your state assemblyman or state senator.

The following steps are recommended by the Public Citizen Health Research Group for individuals interested in obtaining their health records:

1. **Check the statutes in your state**—Even if your state is one of those having no statute granting access, the states generally have no statutes *denying* access, and hospitals or doctors are always free to grant access if they wish.

2. **Contact the hospital or doctor**—Ask what procedure you should follow, e.g. going in person to the hospital's medical record department or putting your request in writing. If you are refused access, cite the applicable law in your state and make notes of the response.

3. **Submit a written request**—If you have been unsuccessful in obtaining your record, cite the relevant law in your letter and be specific about the part or parts of the record you wish to obtain. (Consult the chart at the beginning of this chapter; the most useful documents to you are likely to be the Discharge Summary, Operative Report and X-Ray Reports.) The hospital may charge you a fee for these copies. Keep a copy of your correspondence.

What to Do if Your Request is Denied

If you live in a state where there is no statute permitting access to medical records and if your request to a provider has been denied, you may consider using the help of patient rights groups in your area. However, the most successful way around this obstacle is to have the hospital release a copy of your record to a physician who will share the information with you. Since you are the "owner" of the information contained in the record, you must be the one to authorize this release. Even this may be unnecessary, since the physician who took care of you in the hospital usually keeps copies of your Discharge Summary, Operative Report and X-Ray Reports with his office records, and will often share these with you even if not required to do so by law. Failing this, you may wish to have your lawyer make a request for your records in your behalf. The last resort, of course, is to sue the health care provider. The other course of action is to work toward passage of an access bill in your state.

Access to Records in Federal Facilities

Under the Privacy Act of 1974, patients in Veteran's Administration hospitals, Public Health Service hospitals, or military hospitals have the right to inspect, copy, and correct information in their medical records. You should first telephone the hospital to determine the procedures you should follow. You may be required to submit a written request. If for any reason you are unable to obtain these records, you should write to:

Freedom of Information Clearinghouse
P.O. Box 19367
Washington, D.C. 20036

Obtaining Copies of Your X-Rays

X-rays performed in the hospital or physician's office are a valuable record of the course of your IBD. They are often required for comparison over the years of illness and treatment. Hospitals and physicians are required by law to keep x-rays for a period of time (as defined by state law). After this time period, x-rays are either destroyed or sold to retrieve the silver content of the film itself. Before they are destroyed, or at any time, you may request that a copy be made (at your expense). Many physicians will simply give these older x-rays to their patients as a record of treatment. Together with the written hospital or office record, x-rays enable a person with IBD to have a basic understanding of the course of IBD treatment.

Understanding Your Records

The medical record contains many words and abbreviations which you may not understand at first. This medical terminology, medical jargon, or "medicalese," as it is often called, is a kind of universal convenient shorthand used by physicians, nurses, and all other health care workers to communicate quickly about the patients they care for. While you can easily look up any terms or words you don't understand in any good medical dictionary, you may have more trouble deciphering the abbreviations you will encounter.

Listed below are some of the most common abbreviations and the parts of the chart where they are likely to appear.

History and Physical Examination

ABD–abdomen
CC–chief complaint
CD–Crohn's disease
Dx–diagnosis
EENT–eye, ear, nose, and throat
BP–blood pressure
BM–bowel movements
GB–gallbladder
GI–gastrointestinal
HEENT–head, eyes, ears, nose and throat
H & L–heart and lungs
H & P or HPE–history and/or physical examination
Hx–history
KLS–kidney, liver and spleen
LLQ–left lower quadrant (of abdomen)
LUQ–left upper quadrant (of abdomen)
NAD–no apparent distress
NSR–normal sinus rhythm (of the heart)
O–eye
O2–both eyes
P & A–percussion and auscultation (techniques for examining the abdomen and thorax)
Palp–palpation (of organs in the abdomen)
RLQ–right lower quadrant
RUQ–right upper quardant
Rx–medications
SB–small bowel
TPR–temperature, pulse and respiration
Tx–treatment
UC–ulcerative colitis
WNL–within normal limits
VS–vital signs
WD/WN–well-developed and well-nourished

Laboratory and Diagnostic Tests

Alb–albumin
BE–barium enema
Cath–catheter
CBC–complete blood count

C & S—culture and sensitivity (tests for bacteria in blood and urine samples)
CX—chest x-ray
ECG—electrocardiogram
EN—enema.
ESR—erythrocyte sedimentation rate
Ex—examination
Fx—fluoroscopy
Hb, Hgb—hemoglobin
Hct—hematocrit
IVP—intravenous pyelogram
RBC—red blood cell
SMA-12—automated test of blood chemistries
TIBC—total iron binding capacity
UGIS—upper gastrointestinal series
US—ultrasound
WBC—white blood cell

Physicians' and Nurses' Orders
(many of these abbreviations stem from Latin terms)

AC—before meals (*ante cibum*)
BID—twice a day (*bis in die*)
c̄—with (*cum*)
HS—hour of sleep (*hora somni*)
IM—intramuscular
IV—intravenous
NPO—nothing by mouth (*nihil per os*)
PC—after meals (*post cibum*)
PO—by mouth (*per os*)
PRN—as needed (*pro re nata*)
QD—every day
q4h—every four hours
QOD—every other day
R/O—rule out
s̄—without
SOS—when necessary (*si opus sit*)
STAT—immediately
TID—three times a day

For Further Information...

Annas, George J., *The Rights of Hospital Patients*. New York: Avon Books, 1975.

Sarath, Maria; Auerbach, Melissa; and Bogue, Ted. *Medical Records: Getting Yours*. Washington, D.C.: Public Citizen Health Research Group, 1980.

16

Dealing With Discrimination On The Job And At School

Most people with IBD don't want to think of themselves as disabled. The word "disabled" suggests a person who is confined to a wheelchair, or someone who is blind or has lost a limb. Yet, when Crohn's disease or ulcerative colitis limit our ability to attend school or report to work regularly, both illnesses can sometimes become handicapping conditions. Thinking in terms of disability is useful because it makes us familiar with laws that have been enacted to protect the disabled, and makes us aware of how these same laws might also protect the person with IBD.

The 1973 Rehabilitation Act was the single most powerful civil rights protection for the disabled ever enacted into law in this country.

Gains for the Disabled

Fortunately, Americans with many different kinds of disabling conditions—the physically and emotionally handicapped as well as the chronically ill—have benefitted greatly from protective laws passed during the 1970's, rightly called the "decade of disability." Thanks to lobbying efforts, demonstrations, protest marches and sit-ins by disability rights groups—tactics learned from the civil rights movement a decade earlier—Congress passed the 1973 Rehabilitation Act (Public Law 93-112). Section 504 of this law deals with non-discrimination under federal grants and reads:

> "No otherwise qualified handicapped individual in the United States shall, on the basis of his/her handicap, be excluded from participation in, be denied the benefits of, or be subjected to discrimination under any program or activity receiving federal financial assistance."

This act was the single most powerful civil rights protection for the disabled ever enacted into law in this country. Simply stated, Section 504 prevents employers receiving federal monies (or those doing at least $2,500 in business with the federal government under Section 503) from refusing to hire the disabled, if reasonable accommodations can be made, and if the disability does not impair the performance of the job. It also means that such employers may not require pre-employment physical examinations. Any questions about disability are barred until an individual has been hired. The sweeping language of Section 504 also offers protection of the disabled in the public schools, in higher education, and in virtually all segments of American life which benefit from federal assistance. (The effects of Section 504 on education will be discussed later in this chapter.)

Applying the Law

Under the 1973 Rehabilitation Act and subsequent regulations issued to ensure its enforcement, a handicapped individual is defined as any person who has a physical or mental impairment that substantially limits one or more of that person's major life activities, has a record of impairment, or is regarded as having an impairment.

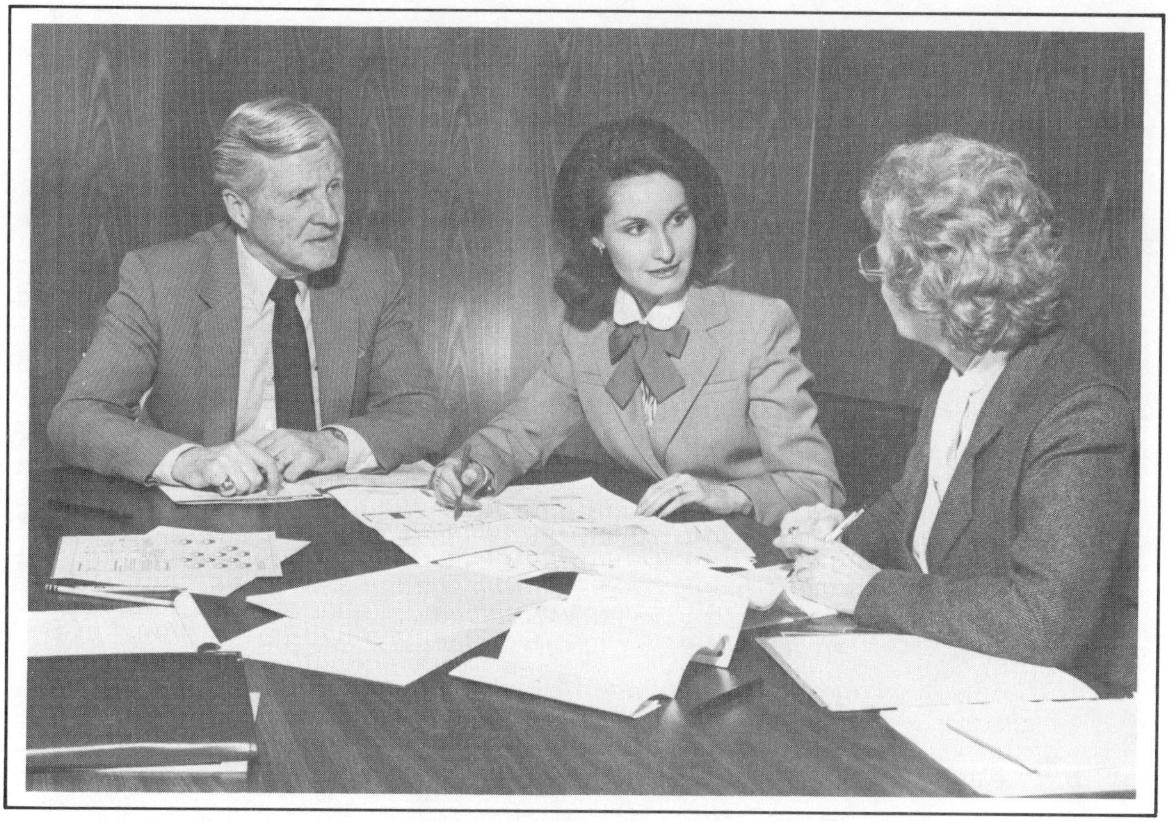

In the application of the law to actual cases, this has meant that a Chicago man's deafness, although a disability, did not prevent him from lifting heavy equipment at his factory job, and that a Texas woman's speech impediment was not a valid reason for her being fired from her job in a bottling plant. It has also meant that a state police academy in Michigan must administer an admission test to an applicant with a history of epileptic seizures. But what does it mean for a person with IBD?

Because IBD has no outward identifying signs, under most circumstances no employer needs to know if an employee has this or any other chronic condition, as long as he or she is qualified and able to do the job. This is also the case if the employee has an ostomy. (Remember, an ostomy is *not* an impairment and should not in any way affect your ability to function at work. In the case of ulcerative colitis, the ostomy, preceded by removal of the colon, has permanently removed the disability of illness.) A person with active IBD may need more frequent access to a bathroom. If this need to use the bathroom facilities does not prevent him/her from completing work assignments, this would seem to be an example of a "reasonable accommodation" which an employer can make under Section 504. Another reasonable accommodation might be the staggering of work hours. Since persons with IBD often experience difficulties and discomfort in the early morning hours, beginning work at 9:30 and ending at 5:30 may make it easier to work a full day. However, if frequent illness-associated absences or stays in the hospital interfere with work performance, the employee may have to negotiate time off and/or a change in responsibilities with the employer. These circumstances are not protected under Section 504.

Editors' Note

The important point is that merely *having* a diagnosis of IBD is not a valid reason for any employer covered by Section 504 not to hire you or to fire you once you have been hired.

Do's and Don'ts for the Working Person with IBD

- Keep the best work record possible. Remember that your employer pays your health insurance premiums as well as your salary.
- If any sick days are necessary, make sure they are documented by a physician's note, not just a "no show."
- Don't ever use your sick days for vacation. You may need them later in the year.
- Keep your illness to yourself. The job is not the place to impress fellow workers and your supervisor with how sick you can be.
- Try to look well no matter *how* you feel.
- Use your break time and meal time wisely—for healthy meals.
- Don't flash your IBD medicines on the job. Keep it professional and private.
- Be honest with your supervisor and boss. If you get sick, warn them and give probable dates of return to work. This will allow them to plan for your absence.
- Use your health care benefits wisely so that your job and your benefits will be there when you need them.

Protection Under State and Local Laws

Protection under Section 504 of the Rehabilitation Act extends to virtually all state and local governments, schools, hospitals, health clinics, social service agencies, colleges and universities, since these are all the beneficiaries of federal funds. But private businesses and corporations, if they receive no federal monies, are *not* required to comply with Section 504. Fortunately, most states have enacted Fair Employment Practices (FEP) laws which cover small businesses (even those with only one or two employees) which are exempt from the federal law. Each year an increasing number of states are expanding the scope of their anti-discrimination laws to protect the employment rights of handicapped persons. Here are some examples:

- **California**—bans job discrimination against individuals with any physical or health impairment. California also makes it unlawful for employers to discriminate against recovered cancer patients.

- **Connecticut**—prohibits discrimination against those with physical disability or mental retardation (if the employee is otherwise qualified).

- **Florida**—bans discrimination on the basis of physical disability, unless the disability prevents satisfactory performance of the work involved. Florida also makes it unlawful to fire or refuse to hire an individual solely because he/she has the sickle cell trait.

- **Hawaii**—bans discrimination against the physically handicapped, and defines physical handicap as a substantial physical impairment that appears reasonably certain to continue throughout the lifetime of the individual.

- **Maryland**—makes it illegal to ask job applicants questions about physical, psychological, or psychiatric illness, disability, handicap, or treatment, unless questions are directly related to job performance. However, medical examination can be required.

- **New Hampshire**—prohibits discrimination in employing the physically or mentally handicapped if these handicaps are unrelated to the ability to peform a particular job, and as long as the individual does not present a hazard to himself or others.

- **New York**—prohibits employers, unions, employment agencies from discriminating because of physical, mental, or medical disability, including blindness or the use of a guide dog.

- **West Virginia**—prohibits discrimination against individuals who are "able and competent to perform the services required, even if blind."

Editors' Note

Be sure to check the Fair Employment Practices laws in your city as well as your state. Remember that most states which ban discrimination against the handicapped also prohibit the asking of pre-employment questions which do not involve the nature and performance of the job. This includes most questions about age, race, color, religion, marital status, age and number of children, and most health-related questions.

How to File a Complaint

If you feel you have been discriminated against in Federal employment or by an employer who is affected by Section 503 (federal contractors) or 504 of the 1973 Rehabilitation Act, you should take the following steps:

1. Write to: Disability Rights Center
   1346 Connecticut Avenue, N.W.
   Washington, D.C. 20036

2. To file a complaint, you or your authorized representative should write to:
   Office of Federal Contract Compliance Programs
   U.S. Department of Labor
   Washington, D.C. 20210
   (for Section 503—federal contractors)

   OR

   Office for Civil Rights
   U.S. Department of Health and Human Services
   Washington, D.C. 20201
   (for Section 504)

Include the following information:

1. Name, address, and telephone number.
2. Nature of disability.
3. Name and address of organization which discriminated.
4. Nature of discriminatory action.
5. The date of such action (Complaints must be filed within 180 days).
6. Any additional background information.
7. How the discriminatory action was harmful to the complainant.
8. Description of previous efforts made to resolve complaints.
9. Name and address of person involved in taking discriminatory action.
10. Copies of correspondence or papers substantiating the complaint.
11. Signature of person who has been discriminated against.

Be sure to send this material by certified mail so that you will know it has been received. Remember to keep a copy for yourself.

Education for the Disabled

The 1973 Rehabilitation Act has also paved the way for full access to education for children with physical, emotional or medical impairments. In 1975, Congress passed the Education for All Handicapped Children Act (Public Law 94-142), requiring a free, public education for all children with a disability. The law contains strong incentives for the states to comply, namely the threatened loss of millions of federal dollars in aid to education. In addition, this legislation has created a climate in the schools where non-disabled students and teachers will gain an understanding of what it means to be disabled through increased exposure to students who are "mainstreamed" into their schools.

For the student with IBD, this means that there is increased leverage for the accessibility of school bathrooms, and that the public school must provide home or in-hospital instruction at no cost to the parents when a child with IBD is too ill to attend school. While these laws will not erase overnight the insensitivity to physical and medical disability found in so many schools, they should give students and their parents the confidence to press for what are now their clear legal rights.

It is still important for the student and his/her parents to assist teachers and school personnel in understanding how best to address the particular problems IBD poses for the student. NFIC's brochure, "A Teacher's Guide to Crohn's Disease and Ulcerative Colitis," was specifically developed to accomplish this purpose.

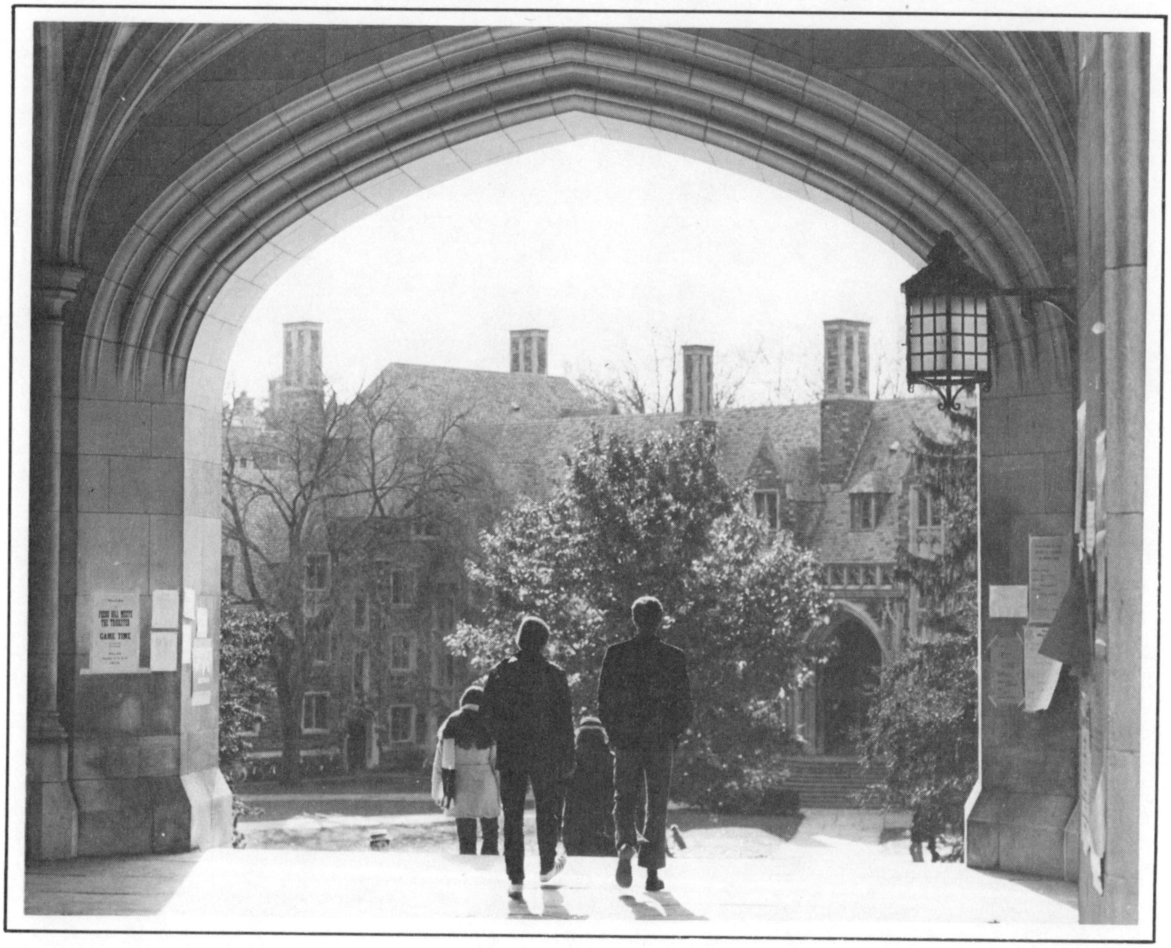

Access to Higher Education

Section 504 and the Education of All Handicapped Children Act broke new ground in higher education as well, assuring non-discrimination in admissions, placement, housing, financial aid, and in all aspects of student life at colleges and universities. Under Section 504, college and university publications, brochures, and applications must contain a statement of nondiscrimination on the basis of handicap in the recruitment and admission of students. Inquiry about a physical or medical impairment may be made only *after* admission of a student. Medical information can be solicited, for example through a medical examination, after an applicant has been admitted if the medical information obtained is not used for the purpose of excluding or disqualifying anyone who is qualified to participate in any of the institution's programs or activities.

The student with IBD who is applying to college should remember that under Section 504, he/she is *not required* to reveal any information about the facts or history of his/her illness. This applies as well to those persons sending letters of recommendation in the student's behalf. However, under certain circumstances, it may be advantageous for the student to disclose the fact of his/her illness, for example when high school grades have suffered because of time spent in the hospital. A letter from the student's physician stating the facts should alert the admissions office to the reasons for long absences from school and the potential medical needs of the student while on campus. However, under Section 504, it is the responsibility of the interviewer or admissions officer *not* to use this information about the student's medical impairment to influence decisions about admissions.

Section 504 also requires that student orientation programs must be accessible to all students. Some colleges and universities have adopted the practice of holding week-long orientation sessions for freshmen in a camp setting where there is little or no access to toilet facilities. Needless to say, this type of situation presents enormous problems for the students with IBD, who may choose to avoid the orientation altogether. College officials may need some further prompting from parents as to what constitutes an impediment to full participation in college life. Again, the student with IBD and his/her family must take the lead.

If you feel that you have been denied admission to a college or university or have not been permitted to participate fully in campus life on the basis of your handicap (medical impairment), you or your authorized representative should file a written complaint with the college or university. The complaint should explain:

- Who was discriminated against.
- In what way.
- By whom of which institution.
- When the discrimination took place.
- Who was harmed by the discriminatory act.
- Who can be contacted for the information.
- Your name, address, zip code and telephone number.
- As much background information as possible.

If you are not satisfied with the response you get, file a written complaint with the Office for Civil Rights, Department of Health and Human Services, Washington, D.C. 20201.

For Further Information...

The College Guide for Students with Disabilities, by Elinor Gollay and Alwina Bennett. Contains information to assist students who have any type of disability which requires special accommodation, information about college policies toward students with disabilities, as well as information about specific types of support services available. Abt Publications, 55 Wheeler St., Cambridge, MA 02138.

17

Paying For Your Health Care: An Update On Health Insurance

With health care costs continuing to rise at a pace well above the national inflation rate, all Americans should be afforded the opportunity to purchase adequate medical coverage. Such coverage could well determine whether or not a catastrophic illness forces an individual or family into bankruptcy. Since the United States, unlike most industrialized nations of the world, has no national health insurance program covering all its citizens, 75 percent of Americans (according to a recent Census Bureau study) rely on Blue Cross/Blue Shield plans or on private health insurance plans, most of them obtained through the work place. This presents a series of potential dilemmas for people with chronic illnesses like IBD:

- They must rely on a health insurance system which places them in a high-risk category or excludes them altogether.
- They cannot be sure they will always be well enough to work.
- They risk losing medical coverage when they can no longer work.

Having a chronic illness in an economic system which favors the healthy makes it essential to know all the possible options for obtaining health insurance coverage. This chapter provides a review of currently available options for the person with IBD.

How Does Health Insurance Work?

The Blue Cross plans in effect throughout the U.S. evolved as a way to insure that groups of patients would be able to pay their hospital bills. Today, each Blue Cross association negotiates a separate contract with each hospital in the community and reimbursements for hospital care are made directly to the hospitals. Blue Shield plans are agreements between the local Blue Shield association and the individual physician or group practice in which the physician receives all or part of the fee for service from Blue Shield.

Private or commercial insurance companies such as Prudential, Aetna, or Metropolitan Life are in the health insurance business for a profit. They make money by insuring as many healthy people as possible and by excluding or limiting coverage for people with chronic illnesses. Your premiums (usually paid by your employer) buy a set dollar value of health related service, e.g. hospital days, office visits, x-ray examinations, etc., and payments are made directly to you to assist you in paying these bills.

Because people with IBD and other chronic problems do cost more for hospital and office care than do healthy individuals, the person with IBD is usually considered a high risk to an insurer.

Because people with IBD and other chronic problems *do* cost more for hospital and office care than do healthy individuals, the person with IBD is usually considered a high risk to an insurer. However, since most companies offer group health benefits through employers, the liability of carrying a high risk employee is spread over a larger group of healthy employees. This makes it possible, in most cases, for a working person with a "pre-existing condition" like IBD to obtain group coverage. Premiums for this coverage are usually paid by the employer, although some companies may require co-payments from employees.

Fortunately, most individuals with Crohn's disease or ulcerative colitis are healthy enough to work at regular jobs, or are covered as dependents under the health insurance policy of a family member. But even those who *are* working may find that the policy offered by their employer does not cover pre-existing conditions until after a full year of employment, or will cover them only after a fixed period of time during which they are "symptom-free" or "treatment-free."

It is also generally true that the larger the company or institution you work for, the more generous the medical coverage is likely to be, and, in most cases, the fewer the restrictions in covering persons with chronic illness like IBD. Conversely, a smaller company may offer a less comprehensive (and less expensive) medical insurance policy with more restrictions. If it is at all possible to choose, the individual with IBD who needs good medical coverage would do far better working with a large employer. In any case, be sure to ask about medical benefits *before* you are hired.

What Kind of Health Insurance Coverage Should I Have?

A good health insurance plan for the person with IBD will offer the maximum number of in-hospital days (usually 120 or 365) in a semi-private room per year. (As a lesser alternative, some commercial carriers offer to pay a flat amount per hospital day or to pay the entire cost after the first $1,000 you pay.) The major medical portion of your coverage should cover physician fees in the hospital. Some plans pay after the first $100-$200 or more deductible, and some offer co-payments for physician charges.

It is important to check whether your plan covers out-patient procedures such as endoscopy and diagnostic x-rays. While in the past, some insurance carriers refused to pay for out-of-hospital testing, these tests are increasingly being done out of the hospital to contain costs.

Coverage for office visits to the physician of your choice is also extremely important to you. Unfortunately, many plans do not pay for these unless they are diagnosis-related. This is fine for your IBD visits to your gastroenterologist, but not for routine primary care.

Conversion to Individual Medical Coverage

If you are leaving employment and have not yet found your next job, find out if you can convert your group medical coverage to an individual plan for which you pay the premiums. In many instances, Blue Cross plans will not enforce restrictive "pre-existing conditions" clauses if your coverage with them has been continuous. If you can arrange for this type of conversion, *pay your premiums promptly and regularly!* If you allow your individual insurance to lapse, you may not be able to obtain coverage again unless you begin working again.

Other Options for Coverage

If a group plan is not available to you at work, or if you are unemployed or unable to work, youwill have a *very difficult time* obtaining medical coverage. If you find yourself in this situation, there are a few options you might explore. In some states and cities, Blue Cross/ Blue Shield offers an "open enrollment period" for a few weeks of each year. During this time, they will accept applications for individual coverage from people desiring medical insurance. If this option is available in your state, *you should take advantage of it* even though the premium will be relatively high. It wil be your *only available* medical coverage and it is always possible to convert to group coverage should you begin working again.

No matter what type of family plan you have, the most important thing is to insure continuous coverage for your son or daughter with IBD before he or she reaches the upper age limit.

A second option which you should explore is the group medical coverage frequently offered by fraternal organizations, clubs, national associations, etc. Because of their large membership, these organizations can sometimes offer low-cost group medical insurance to paid-up members. If you belong to such an organization, you may be able to obtain some medical coverage in this way.

Health Insurance for Your Child with IBD

Coverage for minors under most Blue Cross plans expires at the age of 19. In some cases, the upper age limit is 23. At least one full year before the age limit is reached, parents of a child with IBD should begin inquiring about an individual policy in their son's or daughter's name. If the young IBD patient is a student in college, it may be several more years before he or she is ready for employment, and most student health plans do not have the breadth of coverage necessary for inflammatory bowel disease. Also, because IBD in young people is frequently more severe, many are unable to work and therefore cannot obtain medical benefits on their own.

No matter what type of family plan you have, the most important thing is to insure continuous coverage for your son or daughter with IBD *before* he or she reaches the upper age limit. Most medical plans offered by commercial insurance carriers contain some kind of conversion privilege for the dependent child. Even if this coverage is expensive, *it is far better than no coverage at all*, and can almost always be replaced by group coverage once he or she begins working.

Health Insurance Risk-Sharing Pools

Despite the options to group coverage mentioned above, an estimated one million Americans cannot purchase health coverage because of their pre-existing conditions. Many of these are unemployed or self-employed people with no access to group insurance. Recently, groups of these self-employed people, mainly farmers and ranchers, have enlisted the support of state legislators to establish health risk-sharing pools. These plans vary from state to state but have certain basic features in common:

- All health insurance companies doing business in the state join forces to form an association. The association develops a plan stipulating benefits, including reasonable and customary charges, deductibles, stop-loss, premiums, etc.

- The association then appoints a lead carrier to administer the plan. Individuals are contacted who may meet the eligibility criteria, which are spelled out in the enacting legislation. (This may involve specific requirements such as proof of rejection by a health insurance carrier.)

- The pool then acts as an insurer of last resort for the ill person unable to purchase health insurance in the state.

According to Communicating for Agriculture, a Minnesota-based farmers' and ranchers' association active in lobbying for these risk-sharing pools, plans currently in effect in nine states have provided coverage for more than 12,000 Americans previously unable to purchase health insurance. Legislation to establish risk-sharing pools is pending in an additional 17 states.

States with health insurance risk-sharing pools now in effect are:

Connecticut	Minnesota	North Dakota
Florida	Montana	Rhode Island
Indiana	Nebraska	Wisconsin

Legislation has been introduced to establish pools in:

Arizona	Iowa	Mississippi	Oregon
California	Kansas	Missouri	South Carolina
Colorado	Kentucky	New York	South Dakota
Illinois	Maryland	Ohio	Texas
			Utah

If you wish to learn more about a risk-sharing pool which is in effect in your state, you may refer to the list of contacts below:

Connecticut	Ms. Sandra Downes The Travelers Insurance Company One Tower Square Hartford, CT 06115 203-527-5369
Florida	W.R. Pace, SCHA Coordinator G-15C Larson Building Tallahassee, FL 32301 904-487-2161
Indiana	Ms. Helen Adrian, Deputy Commissioner Indiana Department of Insurance 509 State Office Building Indianapolis, IN 46204 317-232-2418
Minnesota	Mr. Dave Platt, Manager, Underwriting Research and Contracts Department Blue Cross/Blue Shield P.O. Box 64560 St. Paul, MN 55164 612-456-8561
Montana	Mr. Elmer V. "Sonny" Omholt Commissioner of Insurance Mitchell Building P.O. Box 4009 Helena, Montana 59601 406-444-2996
North Dakota	Mr. Bob Carlson 4510–13th Avenue S.W. Fargo, ND 58121 701-282-1235
Nebraska	Mr. Dan Quine Department of Insurance State Capitol Building P.O. Box 94699 Lincoln, NE 68509 402-471-2201

Rhode Island	Contact: State Insurance Department
Wisconsin	Ms. Rosemary Van Susteren P.O. Box 7873 Madison, WI 53707 608-267-2305

For Further Information...

For information about pending legislation in your state, you may contact:

Aaron K. Trippler
National Legislative Public Relations Director
Communicating for Agriculture, Inc.
101 East Lincoln Avenue
Fergus Falls, MN 56537
218-739-3241

Medical Cost Containment Programs and How They Affect You

When Congress passed the Medicare program for older Americans and the Medicaid program for needy Americans in 1965, it had little idea that these programs would become so popular *and* so expensive for the American taxpayer. Over the years various cost containment measures have been attempted, the latest of which is the system of reimbursement to hospitals by Diagnosis Related Groups (DRG's).

In the past under these programs, hospitals were reimbursed for the total length of stay (LOS) the patient needed, plus the cost of medications, tests, etc. A patient's need to be in the hospital was certified by a physician on the hospital staff, based on a review of the circumstances of each hospitalizaton. Recently, the federal government, which finances Medicare, developed a way to reduce Medicare reimbursements to hospitals by grouping together related diseases (DRG's) and establishing fixed lengths of stay for each of 468 DRG's.

The DRG system provides strong financial incentives for hospitals to avoid treating chronically ill people with the potential for long, expensive hospital stays.

Under this system a person with either Crohn's disease or ulcerative colitis who enters the hospital under Medicare has a fixed length of stay of only eight days. No extra days are allowed for medication, treatment of anemia, gastrointestinal bleeding, or for specific IBD complications such as infections or fistulas. Extra time is given only when surgery has been performed, when there is a secondary diagnosis such as diabetes, or when the patient is over 70 years of age.

As you can see, the DRG system provides strong financial incentives for hospitals to *avoid* treating chronically ill people with the potential for long, expensive hospital stays. Likewise, the system discourages the performance of expensive diagnostic procedures which are often required by the patient with IBD.

At this moment, the DRG system affects only hospital stays under the Medicare program, but may be extended to cover Medicaid and Blue Cross reimbursements in the future. Since DRG's and other medical cost containment systems are definitely here to stay, it remains for people with IBD and their physicians to work together to make certain that application of DRG's does not compromise the quality of health care available to the patient hospitalized with IBD. The National Foundation for Ileitis and Colitis has plans to coordinate such an effort at the national level, and will most likely work with other voluntary health agencies to make sure that our voice is heard.

Afterword

The Last 50 Years in IBD: A Long and Winding Trail

Henry D. Janowitz, M.D.

This epilogue to a book devoted to the person with IBD, not to the diseases, is not intended to console the sufferers of these disorders, but to survey what we have all learned along the way in this long winding trail toward the ultimate discovery of cause and cure.

What are my answers to the question put to me everyday by patients, "How can you treat a disease whose cause is unknown and for which there is no specific cure?"

I have two answers to this question. My flippant one, which I ascribe to Oliver Wendell Holmes, Sr., is "The way to live to a ripe old age is to have some chronic illness and take good care of it." My serious answer is that one gets over a serious inflammatory illness of unknown origin just as one gets over a disease of *known* origin, by virtue of the body's own resistance, the defense mechanism of the immune system. The aim of *all* therapy in IBD is to tip the balance in favor of the patient's own defense system.

A useful way to see how far we have come despite the gaps in our knowledge about IBD is to look at where we were 50 or so years ago. Join me, therefore, as an anxious intern going out on the wards of the Mt. Sinai Hospital in 1939. How could we study and diagnose IBD then and what did we have to treat these patients? We depended a great deal on the history of symptoms, examined the stool for blood and pus, looked into the rectum with the rigid sigmoidoscope, and sent the stool off to the laboratory to be sure we had not overlooked a parasite or specific "bug." We had available to us x-rays to do a barium enema and we would take pictures of the remainder of the gut by giving barium by mouth and tediously following its course throughout the small bowel. Not too different from what we do nowadays.

But how could we *treat* the patients in 1939? Not very well and not with many medicines. For ulcerative colitis we could give intravenous fluid and electrolytes, some sugar water but no protein or fats, and very few calories. We treated anemia with blood transfusions; indeed we had so little to offer patients, even if they were not anemic we gave them transfusions, little ones daily, just to pick them up. No worry about AIDS in 1939! If the patient were very sick with ulcerative colitis, we would try to put the bowel to rest by doing an ileostomy, but it didn't seem to work. We were also more daring in very toxic patients by taking out the whole colon but this was more risky, since we had no antibiotics except sulfanilamide and our ileostomies were difficult to manage.

For regional ileitis, the only form of Crohn's disease which we knew of, we were happy to make the diagnosis and tell the patient that the cause of his or her suffering was in the small intestine and not in the head! As for medical treatment, we had nothing except to recommend removal of the areas of the small intestine that were involved. This we did in stages, the first being a bypass of the inflamed area. Some patients felt so much better that we often skipped the second stage of removing the bypassed part, which we have come to regret. Now we make every effort to do so in order not to miss a cancer hidden in the bypassed loop.

Such was the dismal situation a little less than a half century ago. If patients and family are disappointed in our slow progress toward cure of their illnesses, and doctors and researchers are frustrated, consider how far we have come in this arduous search. In ulcerative colitis, we can suppress milder and moderate diseases with corticosteroids, and even induce longer remissions in the severely ill with this class of medicines. If these succeed, we can maintain remission with sulfasalazine. If all else fails, we can cure the disease by removing the colon at the price of an ileostomy. But today's ileostomy is much improved and we now have the option of newer cosmetic operations.

In Crohn's disease, we can improve the patient's lot with sulfasalazine, steroids, antibiotics, and immunosuppressive agents. We can treat the complications of stricture, abscess and fistula surgically by removing minimal amounts of bowel.

For both diseases, we can vastly improve the nutritional status with enteral or parental means. Complete recovery from an operation for Crohn's disease or ulcerative colitis is now the rule in this modern surgical and antibiotic era, not the exception.

Each advance in the diagnosis and management of IBD was hard-won and took time and concerted effort by scores of researchers, clinicians and laboratories. There are no short cuts. Discoveries in IBD, as in all of medicine, depend on both skill and chance, and take time. We have really only known about IBD for less than 50 years of the modern era in medicine. So with our patients we grab at straws, hope for short cuts, and are influenced by fashion. I have seen fashions in diet come and go. Lactose intolerance is not synonymous with IBD and removal of milk and milk products does not always help. The nutritional problems of our patients have called forth a huge cry for nutritional cures, but megavitamins and bizarre diets have led only to disappointment. Acupuncture has had its day. Naturopaths and coffee enemas have lured the unwary.

If something is hidden, the way to find it, I believe, is to have lot of people look for it in a lot of places. Since the founding of the National Foundation for Ileitis and Colitis, a lot of smart researchers are out looking for solutions to our problems in all sorts of places. It is always dangerous to predict, but the answers, when they are found, may turn out to be simple.

IV

Appendix

A

IBD Educational Resources In Print And Film

I. BOOKS AND PAMPHLETS

Source/Publisher	Item	Price	Audience
American Digestive Disease Society (ADDS) 7720 Wisconsin Avenue Bethesda, MD 20814 301-652-9293	"Person-to-Person: About Inflammatory Bowel Disease" (pamphlet)	Free	General
Beaufort Books, Inc. 9 East 40th Street New York, NY 10016 212-685-8588	*The Inside Tract: A Complete Guide to Digestive Diseases* Author: Rubin Goldberg	$13.95 (paperback)	Review of all digestive diseases for the layman, with separate chapters on IBD.
Channing L. Bete Company, Inc. 200 State Road South Deerfield, MA 01371 1-800-628-7733	"About Intestinal Disorders" (a Scriptographic booklet)	Free	General; a very short section on IBD.
Bull Publishing Company Box 208 Palo Alto, CA 94302 415-322-2855	*These Special Children* Author: Katerine F. Jeter, Ed.D.,E.T.	$13.95 (paperback)	Parents of children with ostomies; sensitive treatment and good practical advice on coping with the ostomy experience in children.
Canadian Foundation for Ileitis & Colitis 387 Bloor Street East Suite 402 Toronto, Ontario M4W 1H7 Canada 416-593-2740	"Drug Therapy for Ileitis and Colitis" (pamphlet), To be published, Fall 1985	Free	
	Idiopathic Inflammatory Bowel Disease. Dr. A.B.R. Thomson, Editor. 395pp. Canadian Public Health Association: Ottawa, 1982	$15.00 (paperback)	Written for medical students and the sophisticated layman. Much of the material is highly technical.

	"Information For Teenagers About Ileitis and Colitis" (pamphlet)	Free	Teenagers
	"Paul Has Growing Pains" (pamphlet)	Free	General
	"Psychological Aspects of Ileitis and Colitis" (pamphlet)	Free	General
	"Some Frequently Asked Questions About Ileitis and Colitis" (pamphlet)	Free	General
	"Some More Frequently Asked Questions About Ileitis and Colitis" (pamphlet)	Free	General
	"A Teacher's Guide to Ileitis and Colitis" (pamphlet)	Free	Information about IBD for teachers and school administrators.
	"Ten Facts About Ileitis and Colitis" (fact sheet)	Free	General
Marshfield Clinic 510 North St. Joseph Avenue Marshfield, WI 54449 715-387-5471	"Inflammatory Bowel Disease" (24 page booklet) Author: Kevin Parent, M.D.	Free	General
National Digestive Diseases Education Information Clearinghouse 1555 Wilson Blvd., Suite 600 Rosslyn, VA 22209 301-496-9707	"Ulcerative Colitis" (Information sheet)	Free	General
	"Facts and Fallacies about Digestive Diseases" (Information sheet)	Free	General
	"IBS vs. IBD: Two Very Different Problems" (Information sheet)	Free	General
	"Milk Intolerance due to Lactase Deficiency" (Information sheet)	Free	General
National Foundation for Ileitis and Colitis, Inc. 444 Park Avenue South New York, NY 10016 212-685-3440	*The Crohn's Disease and Ulcerative Colitis Fact Book*. Editors: Peter A. Banks, M.D., Daniel H. Present, M.D., Penny Steiner, M.P.H. New York: Charles Scribner's Sons, 1983.	$15.00 (hard bound) ($40.00 with NFIC membership)	General; clear, layman's explanation of IBD, its complications, treatments, and practical advice on how to cope.

Continued National Foundation for Ileitis and Colitis, Inc. 444 Park Avenue South New York, NY 10016 212-685-3440	"Crohn's Disease, Ulcerative Colitis, and Your Child" (brochure)	Free	Parents of children with IBD.
	"Coping with Crohn's Disease and Ulcerative Colitis" (booklet for children and adolescents)	Free	Children and adolescents
	"Living with IBD"—A 20 page booklet designed to help teenagers better understand and cope with IBD. (Companion videotape also available)	Free	Teenagers and pre-teenagers
	"Questions and Answers about Ileitis and Colitis" (brochure) *Spanish translation: "Preguntas y respuestas acerca de la ileitis y la colitis"	Free	General and Spanish speakers
	"Questions and Answers about Diet and Nutrition in Ileitis and Colitis" (brochure)	Free	General
	"Questions and Answers about Emotional Factors in Ileitis and Colitis" (brochure)	Free	General
	"Questions and Answers about Pregnancy in Ileitis and Colitis (brochure)	Free	General
	"Questions and Answers about the Complications of Ileitis and Colitis" (brochure)	Free	General
	"A Teacher's Guide to Crohn's Disease and Ulcerative Colitis" (brochure)	Free	Especially prepared to help teachers and school administrators understand and anticipate the needs of children with IBD.
Pharmacia, Inc. 800 Centennial Avenue Piscataway, NJ 08854 201-457-8000	"How to Cope with Inflammatory Bowel Disease" (booklet)	Free	New IBD patients; copies distributed to physicians to give to their patients.

Raven Press 1140 Avenue of the Americas New York, NY 10036 212-575-0335	*Inflammatory Bowel Disease: A Guide for Patients and Their Families* Authors: Stephen B. Hanauer, M.D., Joseph B. Kirsner, M.D.	$15.95 (hardcover) $10.50 (paperback)	IBD patients and their families; contains some technical material, but offers up to date essential information for coping with IBD.
Reed and Carnrick Pharmaceuticals Piscataway, NJ 08854 201-981-0070	"Inflammatory Bowel Disease" (pamphlet)	Free	New IBD patients; copies are distributed to physicians to give to their patients.
Charles C. Thomas, Publisher 200 South First Street Springfield, IL 62717	*Ileostomy Handbook: Stoma Care and Management Techniques.* Author: Anita L. Price, E.T.	$29.75	Persons who have had ileostomy surgery; also contains advice on appliance care and skin care.
United Ostomy Association 2001 West Beverly Boulevard Los Angeles, CA 90057 213-413-5510	*Ostomy Quarterly* (Journal)	included with membership or $16.00/year for non-members (4 issues)	Ostomates and prospective ostomates; deals with practical aspects of living with an ostomy.
(Space does not permit a complete listing of UOA literature.)	"So You Have, Or Will Have An Ostomy" (brochure) Author: Carol Norris, Ph.D.	$.50	Written with a light touch, it answers questions about living with an ostomy. Excellent for new patients.
	"Colostomies–A Guide" (32 page booklet) Authors: Edith Lenneberg, ET, and Alan Mendelssohn, M.D.	$4.00	Covers physical facts about colostomies, how they function, their care and management. Also available in Spanish, French and Chinese.
	"Ileostomy–A Guide" (48 page booklet) Author: Linda Gross, ET.	$5.00	Includes illustrations and pictures, with sections about surgery, living with an ileostomy, caring for an ileostomy, problems and what to do, techniques, where to find help, manufacturers and their products and a glossary of terms.

Source/Publisher	Item and Description	Price	Audience
Continued United Ostomy Association 2001 West Beverly Boulevard Los Angeles, CA 90057 213-413-5510	"The Continent Ileostomy" (18 page booklet) Author: Sally-Anne Griffith.	$1.00	Describes the Kock pouch ileostomy, how it is constructed (including illustrations), how it works, who are candidates for the surgery, and some of the aspects of living with this type of ileostomy surgery.
	"Employment of the Ostomate" Reprint of an article by Ed Gambrell from the *Ostomy Quarterly*.	$.50	A discussion of the subject which is helpful to employers.
	"Sex, Courtship and the Single Ostomate" (24 page booklet) Author: Donald Binder	$1.00	Discusses attitudes and anxieties an ostomate might have regarding personal relationships.
	"Sex and the Male Ostomate" (32 page booklet) Author: Ed Gambrell	$1.00	Discusses sex problems that can happen to the male ostomate and possible solutions.
	"Sex and the Female Ostomate" (40 page booklet) Authors: Gordon Dickman and Carolyn Livingston	$1.00	Same as above, for females.

II. Films and Videotapes

Source/Publisher	Item and Description	Price	Audience
Baxter Travenol 1 Baxter Parkway Deerfield, IL 60015 312-948-4550	"Second Chance"– (13 minutes) A film about professional football player Rolf Benirschke's battle with IBD. 16 mm film. (Made with the cooperation of NFL Films.)	Available for Rental	General
Kevin Donovan Films 44 Treat Road Glastonbury, CT 06033 203-633-9331	"Focus on IBD"– Information about IBD for young people and their parents. Patient version: 15 minutes Parent version: 18 minutes Sound-slide program, available in carousel/cassette, Kodak-Caramate, or Telex.	$20.00	Young IBD patients and their parents.

Milner-Fenwick 2125 Greenspring Drive Timonium, MD 21093 1-800-638-8652	"Ostomy: A New Beginning"–Psychological preparation prior to an ostomy for the patient and family.	Available for Rental or Purchase	Ostomates and prospective ostomates.
	"Crohn's Disease"–17 minutes "Ulcerative Colitis"–15 minutes Both films teach the facts about IBD by following the lives of persons with the diseases. Available in all videotape formats and 16 mm film.	Available for Rental or Purchase	Designed for newly diagnosed IBD patients; stresses an optimistic approach.
	"Living with IBD"–(20 minutes) Features two teenage patients and how they cope with IBD, its treatments, and its effect on their social lives. George D. Ferry, M.D., of the Kelsey-Seybold Clinic in Houston, narrates and describes how young patients can help the physician to deliver the best medical treatment for IBD. Available in all videotape formats.	$125.00	Teenagers with IBD and general audiences, school health education programs, etc. (20 page companion booklet available.)

B

A Patient's Bill of Rights

Approved by the House of Delegates of the American Hospital Association. February 6, 1973.

The American Hospital Association presents a Patient's Bill of Rights with the expectation that observance of these rights will contribute to more effective patient care and greater satisfaction for the patient, his physician, and the hospital organization. Further, the Association presents these rights in the expectation that they will be supported by the hospital on behalf of its patients, as an integral part of the healing process. It is recognized that a personal relationship between the physician and the patient is essential for the provision of proper medical care. The traditional physician-patient relationship takes on a new dimension when care is rendered within an organizational structure. Legal precedent has established that the institution itself also has a responsibility to the patient. It is in recognition of these factors that these rights are affirmed.

1. The patient has the right to considerate and respectful care.
2. The patient has the right to obtain from his physician complete current information concerning his diagnosis, treatment, and prognosis in terms the patient can be reasonably expected to understand. When it is not medically advisable to give such information to the patient, the information should be made available to an appropriate person in his behalf. He has the right to know, by name, the physician responsible for coordinating his care.
3. The patient has the right to receive from his physician information necessary to give informed consent prior to the start of any procedure and/or treatment. Except in emergencies, such information for informed consent should include but not necessarily be limited to the specific procedure and/or treatment, the medically significant risks involved, and the probable duration of incapacitation. Where medically significant alternatives for care or treatment exist, or when the patient requests information concerning medical alternatives, the patient has the right to such information. The patient also has the right to know the name of the person responsible for the procedures and/or treatment.
4. The patient has the right to refuse treatment to the extent permitted by law, and to be informed of the medical consequences of his action.

5. The patient has the right to every consideration of his privacy concerning his own medical care program. Case discussion, consultation, examination, and treatment are confidential and should be conducted discreetly. Those not directly involved in his care must have the permission of the patient to be present.
6. The patient has the right to expect that all communications and records pertaining to his care should be treated as confidential.
7. The patient has the right to expect that within its capacity a hospital must make reasonable response to the request of a patient for services. The hospital must provide evaluation, service, and/or referral as indicated by the urgency of the case. When medically permissible a patient may be transferred to another facility only after he has received complete information and explanation concerning the needs for and alternatives to such a transfer. The institution to which the patient is to be transferred must first have accepted the patient for transfer.
8. The patient has the right to obtain information as to any relationship of his hospital to other health care and educational institutions insofar as his care is concerned. The patient has the right to obtain information as to the existence of any professional relationships among individuals, by name, who are treating him.
9. The patient has the right to be advised if the hospital proposes to engage in or perform human experimentation affecting his care or treatment. The patient has the right to refuse to participate in such research projects.
10. The patient has the right to expect reasonable continuity of care. He has the right to know in advance what appointment times and physicians are available and where. The patient has the right to expect that the hospital will provide a mechanism whereby he is informed by his physician or a delegate of the physician of the patient's continuing health care requirements following discharge.
11. The patient has the right to examine and receive an explanation of his bill regardless of source of payment.
12. The patient has the right to know what hospital rules and regulations apply to his conduct as a patient.

C

Chapters of the National Foundation for Ileitis and Colitis

NFIC National Office
444 Park Avenue South
New York, NY 10016
212-685-3440

ALABAMA
Birmingham Chapter–NFIC
c/o Mr. Conrad Cypress
2425 First Avenue North
Birmingham, AL 35203

ARIZONA
Arizona Chapter–NFIC
P.O. Box 37555
Phoenix, AZ 85069

CALIFORNIA
Beverly Hills/Westside Chapter–NFIC
c/o Mr. Ephraim Sales
Wein, Sales & Vizary
8909 West Olympic Blvd.
Suite 200
Beverly Hills, CA 90211

Foothills Communities Chapter–NFIC
c/o Mr. Tom Anderson
1830 Pasadena Glen
Pasadena, CA 91107

Long Beach Chapter–NFIC
c/o Mrs. Elaine Bak
3610 Country Club Drive
Long Beach, CA 90807

Orange County Chapter–NFIC
P.O. Box 4625
Anaheim, CA 92803

NFIC Western Regional Office
2103 Montrose Avenue, Suite B
Montrose, CA 91020
818-249-0212

Palm Springs/Coachella Valley Chapter–NFIC
c/o Mr. Andrew Raschid
475 Winner Circle South
Palm Springs, CA 92262

Sacramento Valley Chapter–NFIC
P.O. Box 19465
Sacramento, CA 95819

San Diego Chapter–NFIC
6035 University, Suite 31
San Diego, CA 92115

San Fernando Valley Chapter–NFIC
c/o Mrs. Etta Schmerler
22110 Victory Blvd., #C-111
Woodland Hills, CA 91367

San Francisco Chapter–NFIC
3216-C Geary Blvd.
San Francisco, CA 94118

COLORADO
Rocky Mountain Chapter–NFIC
c/o Barbara Lanz
1112 East Otero Place
Littleton, CO 80122

CONNECTICUT
Fairfield/Westchester, NY Chapter–NFIC
P.O. Box 1295
Greenwich, CT 06830

New Haven Chapter—NFIC
P.O. Box 9176
New Haven, CT 06532

Greater Hartford Chapter—NFIC
c/o Mrs. Cathy Costa
25 Rosemary Lane
South Windsor, CT 06074

DISTRICT OF COLUMBIA

Greater Washington D.C. Chapter—NFIC
P.O. Box 15402
Arlington, VA 22215-0402

FLORIDA

Ann Gorlitz/South Florida Chapter—NFIC
12550 Biscayne Blvd
Suite 605
North Miami, FL 33181

GEORGIA

Atlanta Chapter—NFIC
554 Monroe Place, N.E.
Atlanta, GA 30324

Central Savannah River Area Chapter—NFIC
c/o Mr. Dennis DiChiaro
426 Halifax Court
Martinez, GA 30907

HAWAII

Hawaii Chapter—NFIC
c/o Ms. Deborah Weiss
47-320-E Hui Iwa Street
Kaneohe, HI 96744

ILLINOIS

Carol Fisher Chapter—NFIC
(North Suburban Chicago)
430 North Merrill Avenue
Park Ridge, IL 60068

Chicago Metropolitan Chapter—NFIC
c/o Mr. Al Dunn
8335 Kostner
Skokie, IL 60076

East Central Illinois Chapter—NFIC
c/o Ms. Linda Rigdon
607 McGregor
Bloomington, IL 61701

Lake County Chapter—NFIC
P.O. Box 793
Libertyville, IL 60048

South Suburban Chapter—NFIC
c/o Mrs. Dorothy Cleary
562 H Aberdeen Road
Prestwick Country Club
Frankfort, IL 60423

IOWA

Iowa Chapter—NFIC
c/o Mr. Ron Popham
RR #1, Box 11
Riverside, IA 52327

KANSAS

Kansas City Chapter—NFIC
c/o Stephen R. Kunz, M.D.
4320 Wornall Road
Suite 128
Kansas City, MO 64111

LOUISIANA

New Orleans Chapter—NFIC
c/o Mrs. Roslyn V. Martinez, R.N.
East Jefferson General Hospital
4200 Houma Blvd.
Metairie, LA 70011

MARYLAND

Maryland Chapter—NFIC
c/o Mrs. Pearl Lewis
6400 Cross Country Blvd.
Baltimore, MD 21215

MASSACHUSETTS

Greater Boston Chapter—NFIC
17 Avery Square
Needham Heights, MA 02194

MICHIGAN

Flint Chapter—NFIC
c/o Mr. Robert Bartelt
11309 Grand Oak Drive
Grand Blanc, MI 48504

Grand Rapids Chapter—NFIC
c/o Ms. Coleen Curtin
448 Cambridge
East Grand Rapids, MI 49506

Michiana Chapter—NFIC
c/o Mrs. Marge Haman
536 Gettysburg Drive
Niles, MI 49120

Michigan Chapter–NFIC
17000 West Eight Mile Road
Suite 238
Southfield, MI 48075

MINNESOTA

Minnesota Chapter–NFIC
c/o Midway Hospital
1700 University Avenue West
Room 301
St. Paul, MN 55104

MISSOURI

St. Louis Chapter–NFIC
c/o Ms. Marla Schorr
2440 Akins Drive
St. Louis, MO 63136

NEVADA

Nevada Chapter–NFIC
c/o Mr. Chuck Giampa
2235 East Flamingo
Suite 107
Las Vegas, NV 89119

NEW JERSEY

Bergen/Passaic Chapter–NFIC
c/o John & Tina O'Neil
377 Saddle River Road
Saddle Brook, NJ 07662

Essex/Morris Chapter–NFIC
c/o Mrs. Helen Klayman
548 Seven Oaks Road
Orange, NJ 07050

Middlesex/Somerset Chapter–NFIC
c/o Mrs. Irma A. Meyer
949 New Dover Road
Edison, NJ 08820

Ocean/Monmouth Chapter–NFIC
c/o Mrs. Rosemarie Golombos
8 Apollo Road
Manalapan Township, NJ 07726

Union Chapter–NFIC
c/o Mrs. Linda Weiss
899 Lambert's Mill Road
Westfield, NJ 07090

NEW YORK

Albany Chapter–NFIC
P.O. Box 1721
Albany, NY 12201

Greater New York Chapter–NFIC
444 Park Avenue South
New York, NY 10016

Southern Tier Chapter–NFIC
c/o Ms. Moya Piros
Binghamton General Hospital
Mitchell Avenue
Binghamton, NY 13903

Staten Island
c/o Ms. Donna Meadowcroft
80 Jefferson Blvd.
Staten Island, NY 10312

Western New York Chapter–NFIC
P.O. Box 224
Williamsville, NY 14221

NORTH CAROLINA

Charlotte Chapter–NFIC
1301 Atando Avenue
Charlotte, NC 28206

Triad Chapter–NFIC
(Greensboro, High Point, Winston-Salem)
P.O. Box 8373
Greensboro, NC 27419

Triangle Chapter–NFIC
(Chapel Hill, Durham, Raleigh)
203 Northwood Drive
Chapel Hill, NC 27514

OHIO

Northeastern Chapter–NFIC
23715 Mercantile Road
Suite 210A
Beachwood, OH 44122

OKLAHOMA

Oklahoma City Chapter–NFIC
c/o Mrs. Julie Costello
420 S.W. 32nd Street
Moore, OK 73160

Oklahoma Chapter–NFIC
c/o Doctors Hospital
2323 South Harvard
Room 236
Tulsa, OK 74114

PENNSYLVANIA

Berks County Chapter–NFIC
P.O. Box 6162
Reading, PA 19610

Lehigh Valley Chapter–NFIC
c/o Ms. Carol Balcavage, R.N., E.T.
Lehigh Valley Hospital Center
1200 S. Cedarcrest Blvd.
Allentown, PA 18105

Philadelphia/Delaware Valley Chapter–NFIC
7718 Castor Avenue
Philadelphia, PA 19152

Pittsburgh Chapter–NFIC
P.O. Box 5445
Pittsburgh, PA 15206

RHODE ISLAND

Rhode Island Chapter–NFIC
P.O. Box 6771
Providence, RI 02940

SOUTH CAROLINA

South Carolina Chapter
c/o Mr. Martin Lefkowitz
2213 Bob White Lane
West Columbia, SC 29169

TENNESSEE

Chattanooga Chapter–NFIC
P.O. Box 80054
Chattanooga, TN 37411

Mid-South Chapter–NFIC
c/o Mr. Maurice Plough
5908 Kermit Drive
Memphis, TN 38119

Nashville Chapter–NFIC
c/o Endoscopy Laboratory
Parkview Medical Center
230 25th Avenue North
Nashville, TN 37203

TEXAS

Austin Chapter–NFIC
c/o William G. Gamel, M.D.
1910 West 35th Street
Austin, TX 78703

Dallas/Fort Worth Chapter–NFIC
2312 Oakland Blvd.
Suite 14
Fort Worth, TX 76103

Houston/Gulf Coast Chapter–NFIC
2650 Fountainview
Suite 122
Houston, TX 77057

San Antonio Chapter–NFIC
c/o Mr. Joseph Slattery
6119 Windy Knoll
San Antonio, TX 78239

VERMONT

Vermont Chapter–NFIC
c/o Mr. Howard Klein
122 Twin Oaks
South Burlington, VT 05401

VIRGINIA

Richmond Chapter–NFIC
P.O. Box 29211
Richmond, VA 23229

WASHINGTON

Puget Sound Chapter–NFIC
P.O. Box 912
Olalla, WA 98359

WISCONSIN

Greater Milwaukee Chapter–NFIC
P.O. Box 13624
Milwaukee, WI 53213

La Crosse Chapter–NFIC
c/o Mr. George J. Italiano
621 Avon Street
La Crosse, WI 54601

Index

A

B

C

D

E

F

M

N

O

P

U

V

W

X

Y

Z

Index prepared by June G. Rosenberg, Information Consultant, Brooklyn, New York